MW01616726

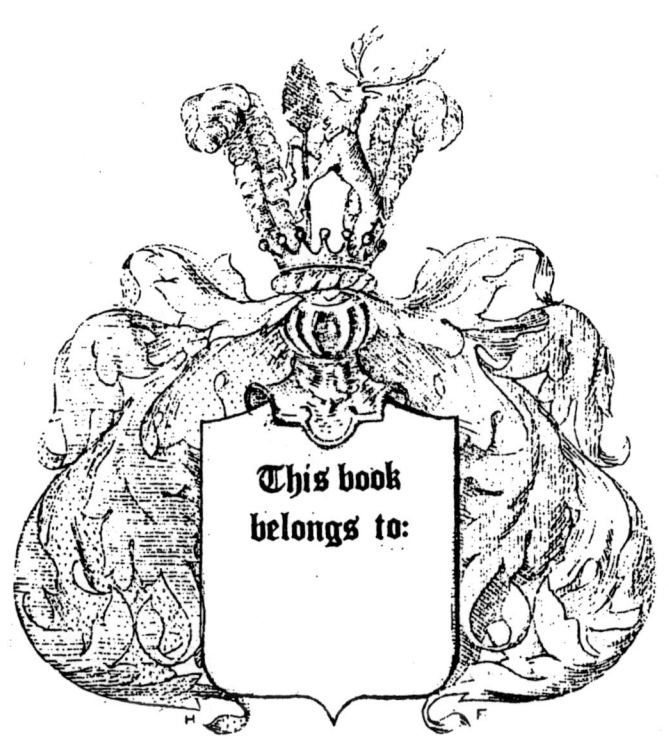

This book
belongs to:

TESTIMONIALS

"I want to show you my gratitude and share my experience ...I came to you with a new fiery outbreak of eczema ... not only the excruciating itching stopped but within 2 days the redness and dryness were completely gone...."
       R. Amendola, designer

"...thank you for your care and guidance regarding my health.... You are an inspiration to me ..."
       J. Mans, editor

"...thank you for all your helpful hints ... you are a true gift from the one above ..."
       G. Grace, performer

"... your book is wonderful ... it is a true inspiration ... you are a living example..."
       D. Garcia, artist

"... the discussion of health can not be complete until I mention you. I am impressed so much by persons who practice what they preach..."
       M.Kosciewicz, author

"...your book has lots of good suggestions, easy to read, and just plain interesting, including the sharing of your personal experiences..."
       M.Hanson, public relations

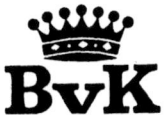

REJUVENATE!

MY HEALTH AND BEAUTY TIPS

Text and illustrations
by

Baroness Benita von Klingspor

The health information and procedures in this book are
based on the training, personal experience, and research
of the author.
Because there is always some risk involved, the author and
publisher are not responsible for any adverse effects or consequences from the use of the suggestion or procedures in
this book.
Please do not use the book if you are unwilling to assume
the risk. Feel free to consult other qualified professionals.

Copyright © 2003 by Benita von Klingspor / BvK
Illustrations copyright © 1985/2003
Baroness Benita von Klingspor

e-mail: books@benitaBVK.com
web-site: www.benitaBVK.com

P.O.BOX 9086, Marina del Rey, CA-90292

All rights reserved.
No part of this publication may be reproduced, stored in a retrieval
system, or transmitted, in any form or by any means, electronic,
mechanical, photocopying, recording, or otherwise, without the
prior permission from the author.

ISBN 0-9721466-1-X

Printed in the United States by Morris Publishing
3212 East Highway 30 • Kearney, NE 68847
1-800-650-7888

10 9 8 7 6 5 4

For Charleen

Acknowledgements

My thanks to Julie Maness
whose editorial assistance was invaluable
in the preparation of this book.

◆

My thanks to Doug Frank
who always helps keep me up to date on
the latest research and products.

◆

Maryann Weaver and Sherry Keaveney
thank you so
for your support and laughs.

TABLE OF CONTENT

Dedication i
Acknowledgements . . . ii
About the author . . . vii

CHAPTER ONE
DAILY HABITS BECOME YOUR PERSONALITY 1
Mirror – Mirror on the wall . . 2
Framework of the body . . 5
Good posture 7
Zwetschgenpopo . . . 9
Don't create your own Dowagers's hump 12
Food and health for bones . . 14

CHAPTER TWO
EYE CARE 19
The eyes reveal your health and soul . 20
Support your eyes . . . 22
Dandelion . . . 25
Milkthistle . . . 25
Bilberry . 26
Lutein 27
The eye-lid work-out from a Princess . 29

CHAPTER THREE
SKIN& & HAIR CARE . . . 33
Read your labels! . . . 34
Is your hair dry and dull? . . 39
Hair treatment from an Empress . 41
'Reversed' hair conditioning . . 45
Home-made conditioners . . 46
The stimulating face scrub . . 49
Smoking – a deadly, poisonous habit . 54

CHAPTER FOUR

PMS & MENOPAUSE . . 57
Good news! 59
Hormone stimulation therapy . . 63
What to wear when trying to reduce . 67
The language of the body . . 70 .
Intestinal cleansing . . . 75
Soy and the thyroid . . . 77
Air conditioning and its detriments . 79

CHAPTER FIVE

YOUR RESTFUL HAVEN . . . 81
Time to start a project. . . 82
Important lessons I learned . . 88
Create a relaxing area - your haven . 90
The low-cost mini-health spa . . 92
The mini-gym 98
Give your closet a face-lift . . 100
First aid supplies . . . 103

CHAPER SIX

BEING A VEGETARIAN . . . 106
Did you know? . . . 113
Green foods 115
Proper pH balance . . . 117
The difference between teas . . 121
How to brew a perfect cup of tea . 125

CHAPTER SEVEN

PHYSICAL MAINTENANCE . . 127
Don't hold your breath! . . 128
The "5-way twist" . . . 129
Various positions . . . 134

CHAPTER EIGHT
ANIMALS HAVE RIGHTS TOO .   .   139

IN CONCLUSION   .   .   .   145

OTHER BOOKS BY BvK .   .   .   147

ORDER FORM   .   .   148

ABOUT THE AUTHOR

A very small photograph, in my English Study book in a German school, paved my path for the future ... I was about eleven at that time. To this day, this small photo remains etched in my mind ... the row of palm trees with the ocean in the background reaching to the horizon ... the title read:
     "Santa Monica, California, USA".

At that time, my mother and I were traveling through Germany – and had to remain there, not by our choice, but because the borders were closed. We found ourselves in a country at war ... World War II.

It was not a joyful time; it was most unstable and rather frightening. Germany was preparing for war. Everything was so different from what I had been used to ... and the comfortable, stable life I had known for so many years, was over.

In addition, my mother, a British subject, and I, with a 'stateless' identification, were not exactly politically correct in a country at war.

As air raids became more intense, and the general living conditions were greatly affected, I was often overwhelmed with a sadness and fear due to the hopeless circumstances. I found myself mentally escaping to those palm trees by the ocean... the place with that beautiful name "Santa Monica" – which I knew nothing about at that time. However, I knew 'deep down' that I would eventually be there, away from all the debris of bombed-out houses, the smell of a destroyed and burning city (including the building we lived in), the loss of most of my class mates, the horrible sound of muffled screams from people who were unable to escape from destroyed cellars. I lived with a fear of the unknown, a lack of joy, but mostly ... a lack of hope.

Three of my school friends also found refuge in that small photo, and we promised each other that we would meet in Santa Monica, after 'the war'.

About ten years later, it was 1953 ... the four of us actually met in a small coffee shop on Wilshire Blvd., close to Ocean Park Blvd. ... where those palm trees were facing the ocean. To this day that view still has a magical affect on me.

So, here I am, fifty years later. In these years I have learned much about this country and myself. The major lesson was, that no matter what the circumstances might be ... they seem to always turn out for the best for me.

After my impressionable experiences, and never giving up in spite of circumstances, and with the special guidance in living a healthful life style ... I find myself writing this book. My friends thought I should name it "VENUS OVER 50" but since this book really includes all ages, not only those who are half a century old and older ... I decided to change the title to a more descriptive one.

I have tried to include what helped me and what I find important to improve and maintain health and spirit, as well as to be able to create a comfortable and peaceful lifestyle, fitting one's budget. I hope that this book will also help those who need encouragement and need a little push to start something new.

x

CHAPTER ONE

DAILY HABITS
BECOME
YOUR PERSONALITY

MIRROR – MIRROR ON THE WALL
FRAMEWORK OF THE BODY
GOOD POSTURE
ZWETSCHGENPOPO
DOWAGER'S HUMP
FOOD AND HEALTH FOR BONES

MIRROR – MIRROR ON THE WALL.

Mirrors were always a fascination to me when I was a small child. I loved to watch the reflections from various angles, but most of all, I was amazed when I discovered that I was capable of creating various grimaces just by changing my facial expression. One day, however, my mother happened to observe me and warned me, that if a 'certain' wind blows, my face would remain <u>forever</u> with whatever grimace I created at that moment. From then on, I did not dare to make faces again, in fear that I would have to live with the results of my newly found amusement!

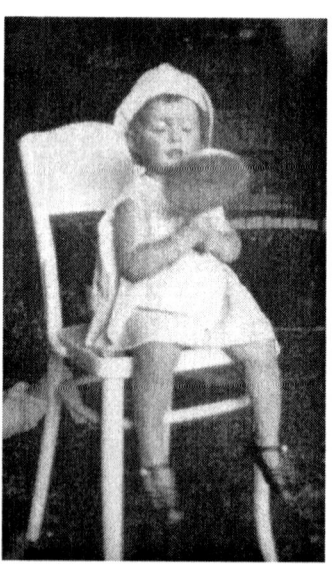

People are often responsible for their own features and posture due to their habits. Facial muscles assume the direction and shape of habitual frowns and expressions, of which one might not even be aware. One of the biggest offenders, I have found ... is negative thinking. It is rather difficult to have a pleasant expression when the mind is filled with unpleasant thoughts. With time, these thoughts can automatically create a harassed, suffering 'lemon-look' which ultimately imprints itself like a map on the face ... just as the growth of a tree is influenced by the direction of the wind ... or better yet, like a work-out program has the ability to affect the muscle tone of the body.

You can help lessen these bad effects by being aware of your thinking patterns and posture. When one carries a heavy load of negative thoughts, the whole body will react to those signals and that can ultimately affect your digestive system, resulting in general health problems, depression, and could include HIGH BLOOD PRESSURE ... your whole image and being can be affected.

Oh, and one more thing ... even a seemingly unimportant habit like not holding your head up straight, could eventually develop into a short-chin-line, which can, as one matures, evolve into a dreaded double chin.

As you can see, poor health habits, if not corrected at a very early age, can influence your whole image, lifestyle and health. It is important, however, to be consistent when one replaces non-supportive habits with beneficial ones which will support you throughout your life ... <u>a discipline which becomes the foundation for a new way of life.</u>

One of the many 'guidelines' I was brought up with, was the importance of looking one's BEST **(for oneself)** at all times. This applies especially when one does not feel well mentally or physically. It might take a little more effort to make a few improvements in order to face the world, but believe me, it is well worth it.

FRAMEWORK OF THE BODY

As a child in Czechoslovakia, I remember seeing people with large humps on their backs. Aware of my concern, my mother explained to me that these people were destined to become angels and that under the hump were wings that had not fully developed, but once they learned how to walk straight and gracefully, their wings would grow and they would be able to fly away.

At the age of four, this made an enormous impression on me, as my greatest wish then was to become like an angel. Even though my mother's story was a bit far-fetched, at the time I believed every word of it and it left me with a permanent visual impression ... **the importance of good posture!**

Little did I know then that those humps were visible evidences of poor carriage, poor nutrition, poor assimilation ... resulting in **OSTEOPOROSIS.**

I think of the body as a container, holding the organs in place with the help of the skeleton ... just like a building with all its rooms which are held together by a strong foundation and framework. If, however, these are inferior, obvious costly problems occur. If the skeleton is deformed due to bad posture from faulty sitting, standing, walking, and due to an unhealthful diet and poor supplements, the internal organs and the skeleton suffer and can't function to their intended potential ... and **you are out of shape!**

You must correct this before it is irreversible, as there is a point of no return! If you are experiencing the results of your bad habits, at least impress this knowledge (the bad and the good) on your children and grand-children, so they will be able to enjoy good health. Schools these days do not seem to emphasize the importance of good form while sitting, walking and eating. They may over-emphasize the competitive values in sports, while neglecting the elements of being in good shape and having good posture.

GOOD POSTURE

The schools I attended in various countries had definite rules aiding good posture. Sitting straight and walking erect were stressed daily. In Czechoslovakia, in the first two grades, we had to sit with our arms crossed behind our back. In Austria, in the third grade, arms had to be folded in front and visible at all times. Slumping was not permitted. In Germany, fourth grade, sitting erect with 4 fingers of each hand on the edge of the desk and the thumb under the desk top ... and of course no fidgeting. Up to the age of 14, schoolbooks had to be carried in satchels on our back to induce good posture. Gymnastics for exercise and grace, the rules of good health, and the knowledge of basic good nutrition were all part of our daily school program.

At the age of ten (or even sooner) we had to participate in gymnastics and calisthenics every day in school and were automatically enrolled in the '*Jahn Turnverein*' where we were taught in more detail about posture, grace and how to strengthen our body.

In order to see our improvements, several times a year, we had to stand one at a time in a wooden open square frame. A cord with a lead weight hung from the top of the frame. As we stood next to it, the teacher could determine if we had correct posture.

I had my first lesson in posture when I was about one year old. I was taught to concentrate on holding the candle straight so the wax would not spill, and not to get my head too close to the flame. This automatically made me walk straight – as you can see in this photo.

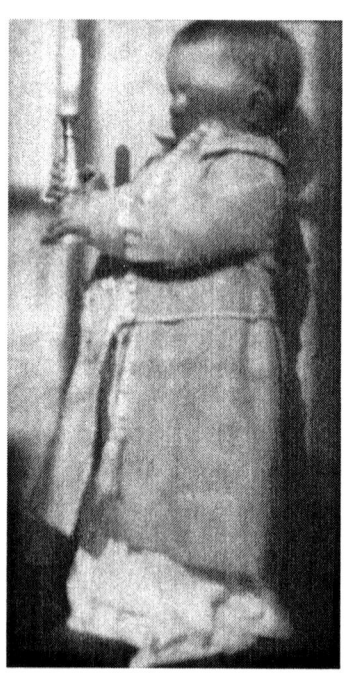

These various rules might sound strict compared to these days, but this part of my daily
schedule really paid off for me.

Good posture should start early in life and
should be part of a healthY habit-forming
lifestyle. After all, one supports a young tree
in order for it to grow straight ... shouldn't this
attention also apply to the growth of a small
child? Slumping and not walking straight will
eventually affect the digestive system ... it
causes the intestines to be 'crushed' - like a
badly packed suitcase.

And while we are on the subject of walking
and sitting straight ... here is another bit of
information you might find interesting.

Beware of the **'ZWETSCHGENPOPO'** ... which
is simply an Austrian term for 'plum bottom'.
Well, I certainly did not want to get stuck
with one of 'those' ... if I could help it. So,
this is what I was directed to do.

Simply sitting straight is not enough. If one
sits down tucking 'it' under, especially if one
has to sit a lot, this will create a flat 'bottom'
and a crease which is not very attractive. To
prevent this, one should sit to the back of
the chair and then slide forward just about

one or two inches. This will help shape the curve by not 'squishing' it and also prevent the crease from developing. It is sort of like 'contouring' your bottom.

So there you have it ... the fight against the 'Zwetschgenpopo' ... it works.

Here is another guideline I was brought up with ... which helps in walking straight and gracefully. This is where visualization helps!

Imagine a string tied to the top of your head with someone pulling the string straight up, like a puppet ... and walk with that image in mind. Try it, it actually helps one's posture and creates a feeling of walking more light footed.

As you can see, I received all sorts of direction ... what slipped past my parents, my governess was sure to catch. But most important ... I gained a great deal from all these guidelines.

These days, 'Pilates' (the floor exercises) have become very popular, which in fact is **calisthenics.** The actual floor technique was not originated by Joseph Pilates. It was part of an organized technique originated by the

'*Jahn Turnverein*' in 1811 ... which to this day is still a well known athletic club throughout Germany. Calisthenics are simple gymnastic exercises, teaching the art of developing bodily strength with gracefulness.

Mr. Pilates was born in Germany in 1880 and also had to participate in this strict regimen. He eventually brought it to England with added equipment ... and it progressed from there.

I try to incorporate various movements into a stretching exercise ... throughout the day. Whether it is reaching for something, bending down, or, ... simply combing my hair.

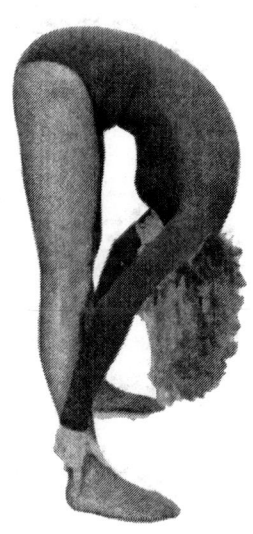

Every morning, I stretch and then bend down, as shown in the photograph . At first this is mainly to flex my body ... my hair hangs freely, blood rushes to my head ... a perfect time to use a wide-spaced brush ... which helps brush and massage my scalp and hair at the same time. A few strong strokes gives a great tingly feeling to the scalp.

DON'T CREATE YOUR OWN 'DOWAGER'S HUMP'!

This bulge at the base of the neck, on many women, has become so accepted as 'part of growing older', that manufacturers of women's clothing adjust certain large pattern sizes accordingly.

You can actually help prevent this hump from forming or progressing by re-shaping yourself, by correcting your posture and by adding mineral supplements to a healthful diet ... and with the assistance of a helpful 'posture tool'.

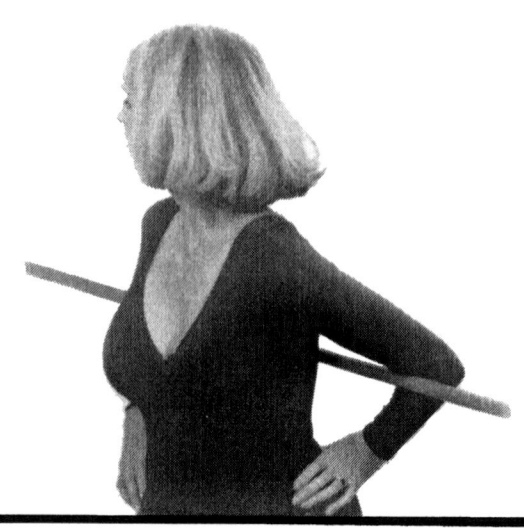

I call it the 'posture-wand'. When used several times a day, it will help in correcting or guiding your posture. You can use a broomstick handle, shortened to about 30 inches, or, buy a one-inch dowel, about 30 inches long.

The exercise is simple: place the stick across your upper back, hold it in place with the upper arms pressing forward. Use this while walking, sitting, or standing. If you twist from side to side, you will also help trim your waistline!

My grandmother used this method daily, no matter where she traveled. She lived 92 years, and the memory of her elegance and graceful posture has always inspired me.

The 'dowager's hump' does not just create a poor visual effect for your posture, it also negatively affects your digestive system and all other bodily functions. When you allow bad posture to be part of your life style, you are actually setting yourself up for eventual physical problems. Just think of how good clothes will look when one walks straight and sits with good posture!

FOOD AND HEALTH FOR BONES

The mineral complex I take, which includes vitamin "D", is right next to my bed, so I won't forget to take it. After all, bones need food too!

Calcium is the most abundant mineral in the body. As you probably know, if you don't get enough calcium, your bones will certainly suffer. When levels of calcium (and other minerals) decline, bones (**OSTEO**) become **POROUS**, brittle, and susceptible to fracture for lack of new bone tissue ... **the rate of bone loss speeds up while the rate of making new bone tissue slows down!** The process of bone thinning is a natural part of aging and cannot be completely stopped.
Bone health, like all living tissue, requires adequate nutrition for proper growth ... and is profoundly affected by our daily food and exercise choices. Although it is best to start during the teen years, adults who follow these habits can prevent or reduce their risk of developing osteoporosis.
Magnesium acts as a catalyst in the system for the vital organs, the heart being the most affected. It is found chiefly in fresh green vegetables, an essential source of chlorophyll! Magnesium deficiency can easily occur because it is refined out of many

foods during processing ... in addition, over cooking foods also removes other minerals and vitamins.

Here are just a few of the benefits when supplementing the diet with magnesium:
It helps prevent leg cramps, muscle weakness, twitching, high blood pressure, and for those who experience constipation ... increasing the amount of magnesium will help with regularity. However, too much of a good thing, could work the other way ... so make sure you take the right amount! Always increase in small segments, until you have the desired result!

It is also essential to add **VITAMIN "D"** – the sunshine vitamin! It helps the body absorb calcium from food, thereby making more of the minerals available to the bones. Consuming more vitamin "D" can slow bone loss and possibly increase bone density ... it may also possibly slow the progression of osteoarthritis, the most common type of bone loss.

Outright deficiency of vitamin "D" prevents new bone tissue from hardening, a condition known as 'rickets' in children, osteomalacia in adults, and clearly worsens osteoporosis ... the brittle-bone disease.

New research indicates that insufficient levels of vitamin "D" are far more common and far more harmful than previously believed. It may weaken the bones, possibly worsen arthritis and perhaps increase the risk of heart disease, diabetes and other disorders.

While too much sunlight can cause cancer ... **our bodies do miss and need sunshine.** The healing centers in Europe use sunshine as part of their therapy. Avoid the burning rays between 11 a.m. and 3 p.m. – when the sun is the strongest ... so, make use of it before or after the strongest rays are present. You could give yourself 10 minutes in the sun <u>before </u>you apply the sunscreen.

SUNSCREEN INHIBITS THE ABSORPTION OF VITAMIN "D"

Also ... other things you can do to maximize your vitamin "D" and calcium absorption ... **eliminate smoking** and **alcohol. Colas** and **root beer** drinks are high in phosphates – which interferes with calcium absorption ... and **caffeine** increases the rate at which calcium is lost in the urine. **They all hinder health!**

As with any supplements, you might check with your physician to make sure these additions will not interfere with any existing medical condition or medications.

In order to support my bones and to avoid degenerative conditions, or at least minimize them, I include the following supplements to my regime ... which I take at bedtime to aid relaxation:

A chelated mineral complex, including
15 mg zinc,
1-3 mg boron,
1 tablespoon silica
400 I.U. vitamin "D"
100 mcg vitamin "K"
1500 mg calcium
750 mg magnesium

Those who are on a high protein diet may put themselves at risk ... high protein leaches calcium from their bones. ... in addition to stressing their kidneys.

My bone density test (at near age 75) indicates that I do not have osteoporosis ... in spite of not drinking milk since being an infant and never having taken part in estrogen re-placement. I credit my healthy bones and my general health to:
♦ calisthenics starting at an early age,
♦ eating and drinking health supporting foods with proper supplements
♦ good posture

NOTES ...

CHAPTER TWO

EYE CARE

THE EYES REVEAL YOUR HEALTH AND SOUL
SUPPORT YOUR EYES
DANDELION
MILKTHISTLE
BILBERRY
LUTEIN
THE EYE-LID WORKOUT FROM A PRINCESS

THE EYES REVEAL YOUR HEALTH AND SOUL

Your eyes need nourishment and relaxation in order to look, feel and perform their best.

If you frown and distort your face to keep the sun out of your eyes, you not only **create wrinkles**, but also give your face an almost perpetual frown ... and you are in the process of creating your future face!

You have probably noticed that when people are looking into the distance, they usually squint. In particular this happens if they are looking toward the sun ...as in looking for the arrival of the bus. This habit is the very beginning of the eventual frown and the dreaded **crows' feet**, and could lead to eventual eye damage.

If your eyes are sensitive to bright light, you might be in need of supplements. Ninety percent of my clients share one symptom in common ... light sensitivity. Most had accepted this condition as normal, and instead of turning to nourishing the eyes, dark glasses have become the automatic choice to combat this deficiency. However, after a few months of taking supplements (depending on the circumstances), great improvements were noticed.

In the 60's, when I found out how risky it is to depend on sunglasses, I tested my colorful collection to see how much ultra-violet light was blocked out by the 'protective' film. At that time I was art director for Hughes Research Laboratories in Malibu ... a perfect place to get advice from the many scientists who were researching that field.

I was shocked to find out that only one pair of the 23 pairs of sunglasses I collected, blocked out UV entirely. It turned out to be the least expensive of them all ... a clip-on-pair by *Polaroid-Land*! However, they do not prevent UV from entering at the sides.

What I learned was rather interesting and made a lot of sense. The eyes are designed to protect themselves from too many UV rays. The pupil will contract and reduce its diameter when exposed to bright conditions, and will dilate or enlarge in conditions of dark surroundings, to gather as much light as possible.

So, if you are wearing dark glasses on a sunny day, you are really giving your eyes the wrong message, which may affect your eyes eventually, if you continue to do so year after year.

Dark glasses are actually helpful if you are in glaring sunlight by water surfaces (pool, beach, etc.), or snow.

According to statistics, California and Florida have the highest rates of eye problems in the elderly. In those states you can certainly find a great variety of dark glasses in any season.

SUPPORT YOUR EYES

One way to help your eyes function better, is **via the liver !** Think of the liver as a bag in your vacuum cleaner. When the bag is full, you will not be able to clean the rug or floor properly. In a way, this applies to the liver as well. The liver has many tasks to perform ... and one of them is ... <u>filtering and cleaning the blood of toxins</u> to better nourish the cells throughout the body, <u>including the eyes.</u>

So in addition to a healthful diet, it's good to support the liver with safe and healing herbs.

During WWII ... our teachers taught us how to help our stressed system to survive the daily and nightly bombing episodes. Among other healthful suggestions, we were told that drinking a tea made of Milkthistle pods and Dandelion would help <u>support the liver and gallbladder function</u>. The whole class had to go out into the fields and meadows to collect the ripened pods of the Milkthistle. The stems and pods have little hairs which stick to anything, especially clothes.

While filling the baskets, we usually ended up having nearly as many pods stuck to our clothes and hair! It was a funny sight and certainly added humor to an unexciting task.

I have been supporting my liver this way for many years and believe that one should not wait until signs of toxicity or damage are felt. In this world of pollution, we are exposed on a daily basis to car exhausts, pesticides, and all forms of other toxic particles. For example, dry-cleaning uses one of the worst chemicals ... it even has an unpleasant odor. For that reason, I only wear clothes made of washable fabrics. Luckily I can sew which makes this an easy choice!

The liver is the largest gland of the body and the only organ that will regenerate itself. Remember, it is greatly responsible to help protect your body from pollutants ... so, why not start now to assist the liver in every way possible. Avoid constipating foods ... the liver has to work twice as hard if you are constipated. Chlorophyll and distilled water with a freshly squeezed lemon are excellent blood purifiers and help liver regeneration. On the other hand, as you probably know, smoking and alcohol consumption are not at all helpful to your liver ... it would be best to eliminate these habits.

Overeating also creates excess work for the liver, resulting in liver fatigue. Remember, when the liver is overworked, it may not be able to detoxify harmful substances properly before they enter the bloodstream ... which hampers necessary nutrients from being absorbed. Don't wait until there is damage, or when it possibly could be too late for your liver to react!

This brings me to **herbs,** which have always been a great part of my upbringing, no matter which country I lived in. In addition, I learned about the harmful and safe ones in the various European schools ... particularly, during WWII. Herbs became a major source of nourishment and healing. To this day, I still include my favorite herbs in my daily routine.

One herb stands out ... **THE DANDELION!**
During the summer, the leaves were always included in most salads ... a great support for digestion. When food became scarce due to the bombing episodes, we were advised to chew the fresh root ... it has many nutrients and is of great support to the liver and gallbladder.

It has the ability to stimulate the liver to detoxify poisons and helps purify the blood, which in turn, helps clear skin blemishes and has proven effective against gallstones and fluid retention.

MILKTHISTLE ... is a detoxifying, rebuilding herb for the liver, with significant anti-oxidant properties to prevent free-radical oxidation.

The active ingredient, Silymarin, which is the active component extracted from the milkthistle, is a flavonoid long recognized in supporting alcohol-induced fatty liver disorders, inflammation of the liver and bile ducts, and hardening of the liver. It has also been found to be beneficial with psoriasis.

Many of my clients have seen considerable improvements in blood tests once the milkthistle was part of their healing program.

In short, the milkthistle is one of the most important herbs and should be a part of your daily intake of supplements.

BILBERRY ... or the European blueberry.
Often our class took trips to the edge of forest areas where blueberries grew in abundance. We were taught about blueberries and how they help strengthen the capillaries throughout the body ... and, since injuries due to shrapnel and debris from bombed areas were a constant threat, we were told to eat blueberries in order to help strengthen the capillaries and support healing in case of an injury.

Now, whenever blueberries are available in the stores ... I make sure to include them in my diet ... they have a somewhat different appearance and flavor than the ones from Europe.

When I noticed 'floaters' in my vision, I increased my intake of bilberry capsules and observed that most of the floaters disappeared after a few months. In addition, I combine bilberry with lutein for more support and feel that this combination has helped me and my clients greatly.

This of course is in addition to a healthful diet at all times.

This brings me to **LUTEIN** ... which plays an essential role in your vision.

I have been supplementing with lutein and bilberry for several years, and even though my close vision was always good, I feel that it became even more clear with this combination. However, when I stopped lutein for about one month because of the lack of availability in Hawaii at the time, I noticed that I was unable to read the very fine print on some vitamin bottles which I usually had no trouble reading. This continued for about three weeks until I was able to purchase lutein again. My vision improved within days and I was able to read the small print on the very same vitamin bottle again. Needless to say, now I make sure that I never run out of lutein. Several of my clients have also noticed great improvement in their vision.

Years ago I read a book by Bill Sardi about eye support. His book and current research supports the fact that increased consumption of lutein-rich foods (kale, collard greens, broccoli, spinach) and lutein supplements increase carotenoid levels in the eyes ... thereby helping to protect them from disease. Research indicates that lutein helps make up what is called the macular pigment in your eye. This is part of the retina that allows you to see straight ahead without distortion, and to read fine print. Research indicates lutein may help maintain eye health and prevent free radical damage in the macula and retina, which are two lutein-rich and highly oxidant-sensitive areas susceptible to age-related macular degeneration (ARMD) and to cataracts. Oxidation and light damage may also cause this macular deterioration. It seems **lutein acts as a natural sunshade**, protecting the eye from too much light. I have to add here, that sun light does not irritate my eyes anymore and I have no need for sunglasses - even though years ago I felt an absolute need for them.

Because eyes gradually lose lutein with age, some researchers theorize that lutein loss leads to retinal sun damage and ultimately to degeneration in macular thickness.

Lutein is truly another very important herb to include in your daily ritual. It is somewhat pricey ... but the results are worth it.

This of course is in addition to a health-supporting pH-balanced diet. It is the simplest way I have found to live, and is easy on the digestive system.

THE EYE-LID WORK-OUT FROM A PRINCESS

Are you concerned about crinkled eye-lids? I have found the following treatment to be of great help, even if only slight symptoms already exist.

Even though my great-aunt, the Princess Zubeida May Djavidan, had a choice of the best skin cares in the world, she used simple techniques to tighten eye-lids.

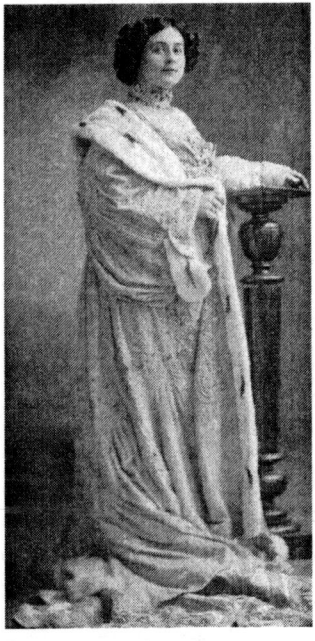

My great-aunt, the Princess Zubeida May Djavidan
At her crowning in 1899, Cairo, Egypt,
when she married Abbas Hilmi II. - the last Khediv of Egypt

I tried her method at the first sign of a crease on the lid ... and to my amazement, I did see a difference within a few weeks. This is what she told me to do ... and this is what I did:

To perform the eyelid work-out, place the side of your index finger firmly, but without pressure, against the bottom of the upper lid while it is open. Try to close the lid while the finger remains in place, making the lid 'work' against it. You will hear a slight sound in your ears, due to the pressure. Do this several times to the count of 5 or more, in the morning and before going to bed. If done daily, this exercise definitely produces results.

This works well for me, since I consider my eyelids as my 'canvas' ... they have to be smooth, so I can brush them with my usual choice of shimmery-golden-bronze powder.

While my great-aunt lived in Egypt and when she traveled, she always made sure that a most dependable remedy was packed in her cosmetic case ... **a raw potato!** She told me that fine slices of potato did wonders for a sunburn and puffiness around the eyes – which at times occurred while riding through the Sahara.

I have often tried this simple method ... and know why she had such good reactions.

Try these most cooling natural rejuvenators:

♦ one medium raw washed **potato**, sliced or, finely grated (like for potato pancakes)
OR,
♦ one peeled, or, finely grated **cucumber**
♦ place a towel under your head, so it will absorb the excess juices while you are lying down
♦ smooth the grated potato or cucumber over your face and closed eyes
♦ leave on for about 10 minutes and RELAX!
♦ after the treatment, remove mixture
♦ wash face with tepid water
♦ apply cocoa butter, or a moisturizer of your choice

In spite of her worldwide adventures and having lived in castles and palaces, my great-aunt eventually decided to settle in a small village outside of Vienna, Austria ... away from her publicized lifestyle.

When I saw her last, she told me that she found great joy in taking care of the flowers in her garden, and painting ... the memories of her past. She lived to be 92.

NOTES ...

CHAPTER THREE

SKIN & HAIR CARE

READ YOUR LABELS
IS YOUR HAIR DRY AND DULL?
HAIR TREATMENT FROM AN EMPRESS
'REVERSED' HAIR CONDITIONING
HOME-MADE CONDITIONERS
THE STIMULATING FACE SCRUB
SMOKING – A DEADLY, POISONOUS HABIT

READ YOUR LABELS!

Decades ago I found this amusing poem, the author was not mentioned ... I thought it would be most appropriate for this chapter.

Listen, and take a warning from
The fate of Clementine,
Who strangely disappeared at the
Precious age of nine.
She filched a preparation from her
Mother's dressing table.
Today there's nothing left except a
Small descriptive label,
Which reads in part:

*"If properly applied, you will succeed
in looking ten years younger - and
Results are guaranteed!"*

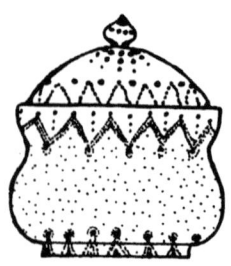

With so many beauty aids available, it is often quite difficult to make a firm decision. However, the ones that claim to make you look years younger ... I question highly! They usually have the ability to tighten the skin for a few hours ... and then what!

Reading labels is important, not only for food items but also for skin care. After all, the skin is the largest absorbent organ, so you should put the utmost care into the selection of what you let your skin take in whether it is soap, shampoo, cosmetics, suntan oil, or lotion. The process of absorption through the skin is particularly important, because it completely bypasses the kidneys and liver, which normally filter out toxins.

I don't suggest that you abandon all the fine cosmetics you have accumulated, but I am sure you might be open to try new combinations.

I have to mention again, the importance of what we eat, drink and absorb, what our habits are and what we think ... these will make a lasting difference on our expressions and health. Also, spending more money does not necessarily assure you that the product is superior, maybe only the jar might be more appealing.

When I select an item, I look for absorption, a slight or no fragrance, cost, free from unnecessary chemicals, and of course:

"CRUELTY-FREE TO ANIMALS".

I concentrate on only a few items:
♦ face & body scrubs that are not 'mushy'
♦ face cream and lotion that absorb well and retain moisture
♦ liquid soap with a pump for hands & body
♦ hair conditioner and shampoo with support for dry, treated and damaged hair. Even though my hair is healthy … these additional ingredients give my hair extra support.

Here are a few items to look out for:

If you suffer from an itchy scalp, you are either not rinsing thoroughly after shampooing, or, your might be allergic to **Sodium _Lauryl_ Sulfate**. It is known to be harsh for some and can cause drying, itching and skin irritations, and stinging of the eyes.

On the other hand, **Sodium _Laureth_ Sulfate,** has been modified and is milder and gentler to skin and eyes. Those with an 'itchy' scalp have felt the difference … but, in addition, rinsing longer is most important.

Following are just a few ingredients you might find in your cosmetics and/or food, (**C** for cosmetics and **F** for food). They are considered safe with no limitations other than 'good manufacturing practices':

ALBUMIN (C & f) ... an emulsifier derived from egg whites. It may cause a reaction to those allergic to eggs. Large amounts can produce symptoms of lack of biotin, a growth factor in the lining of the cells.

CELLULOSE GUMS (C) ... resistant to bacterial decomposition, a mold and yeast inhibitor.

GLYDERYL STEARATE (C) ... an emulsifier, emollient, and humectant.

PHOSPHOLIPIDS (C) ... used in moisturizers, they bind water and hold it in place.

PROPYLPARABEN (C) ... a preservative and bacteria and fungus killer.

CETYL ALCOHOL (C & F) ... an emollient and stabilizer.

CALCIUM CHLORIDE (C & F) ... an emulsifier and texturizer.

PALMITIC ACID (C & F) ... obtained from palm oil ... used as a texturizer.

PHOSPHORIC ACID (C & F) ... made from phosphate rock; an antioxidant ... concentrated solutions are irritating to the skin and mucous membrane.

PROPYLENE GLYCOL (C & F) ... a clear, colorless, liquid to enhance viscosity.

SODIUM BENZOATE (C & F) ... an antiseptic and preservative.

SODIUM CAPRYLATE (C & F) ... also known as PALM OIL.

SODIUM CARBONATE (C & F) ... soda ash. If one is hypersensitive, it could cause scalp, forehead, and hand rashes.

SORBIC ACID (C & F) ... a preservative and humectant, a mold and yeast inhibitor.

STEARIC ACID (C & F) ... occurs naturally in some vegetable oils ... it gives pearliness to hand creams.

IS YOUR HAIR DRY AND DULL?

Continuous visits to beauty parlors are one of
the contributing factors for dry, brittle and
unhealthy hair - even if massages and conditioners are part of your special treatment
program.

Hair is usually put through several processes:
♦ It is first washed ... when the hair shaft
absorbs the shampoo to the fullest, because
the hair was dry at the beginning.
**Shampoo is a cleaning agent, not a nutrient
to support hair.**
♦ After that, it is conditioned while wet, at a
point of no absorption! So you hardly bene-
fit from the extra added treatment which
should support your hair with nutrients!
♦ Then it is rinsed, rinsing most of the expensive
treatment creams down the drain.
♦ Then it is combed while wet, at a time
when hair is in its most breakable state!
♦ After it is set, a hot blower will dry out your
scalp and all the natural oils that give that
healthy sheen and bounce to your hair.
Even if the blower is cool, it still forces the
hair shaft to dry more quickly than when it
dries naturally.
♦ As a grand finale, it gets sprayed with
chemicals to keep your hair 'in shape'.

I am not condemning beauty parlors, but on a weekly basis, this ritual does take its toll on your hair. After all, your beauty operator is guided by a certain time schedule which usually does not include specialized treatments.

If you are concerned about the appearance of your hair, and you and your beauty operator have tried 'everything', add one more method to your long list, and give it a chance to show its results after a few applications. See "HAIR TREATMENT FROM AN EMPRESS" for details. I was brought up with these methods and I continue to use them to this day with the same great results.

Why not incorporate your hair-treatment with your projects at home, on your 'day off', which would usually be spent by driving to and from the beauty parlor ... and not to forget, waiting for your turn plus the actual treatment time!

You will be pleased and amazed to see that by changing just a few steps in the treatment of your hair, it will be easier to manage and you will see the difference after just a few times.

HAIR TREATMENT FROM AN EMPRESS

Empress Elisabeth of Austria-Hungary was known the world-over for her grace, beauty and long, thick hair, which was often braided into the shape of a crown – adorned with diamond clips.

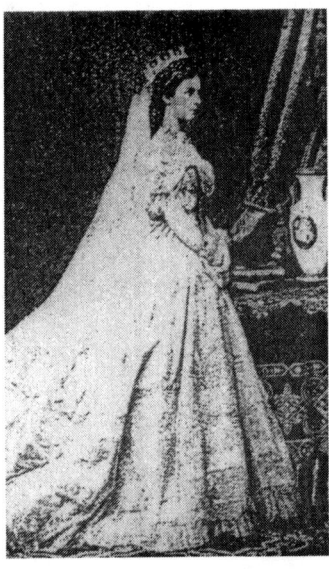

Empress Elisabeth of Austria-Hungary, 1890

From an early age, my mother impressed on me that healthy hair was like a 'crown' and used the Empress as an example of how well taken care of hair should really look. In order to achieve this, I was subjected to special treatments, to assure me of healthy, thick hair in the years to come.

Even though my wish was as a child to have long braids, which I could fling over my shoulders, my hair was kept at ear-length until I was about ten (as shown in photo below). This was to promote thickness, since I had fairly thin hair since birth. I was not exactly overjoyed with that program ... and to partially fulfill my dream, I created braids from wool strings and attached them to my hairclips – pretending to have long, flowing hair.

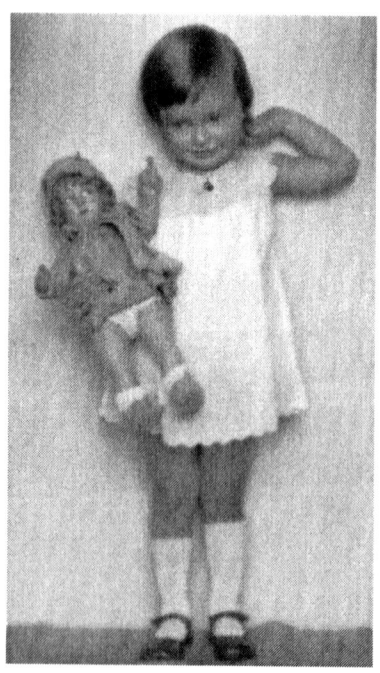

My godmother, the Countess Irma Staray, who was a constant companion to the Empress and who resided at the Austrian court, supplied my mother with various hair treatment recipes which were used for the beautification of the Empress's hair, obviously with great results.

She always stressed that conditioning one's hair is of the utmost importance in keeping it manageable and healthy – especially in the summer. And most important … one should condition **FIRST** … **before shampooing!**

General instructions usually indicate that one should apply the conditioner AFTER one has shampooed or partially dried the hair. At that time the hair shaft does not have the capacity to absorb an additional treatment. Think of the hair like a very thin sponge, it can only absorb a certain amount of moisture. When applying the conditioner after washing, only the outside of the hair will be covered, which is being rinsed off anyway, and you gained very little in this treatment for the amount spent in time and money.

When one conditions the hair FIRST,
before washing … ***when the hair is dry*,**
one supplies essential nutrients to the scalp and hair which can be easily absorbed.

So, when you shampoo your hair first, the shampoo will be absorbed into the scalp and the hair shaft, and will not support your hair with important nutrients to keep it healthy. All it will do ... is clean your hair!

Due to my godmother's suggestion, I always applied the conditioner **FIRST**, when the hair is able to soak it up like a dry sponge ... for <u>maximum absorption and restoration</u>. To this day, my hair is thick and lustrous ... even though I am nearly 75. I am often asked if I am wearing a wig ... and when my clients realize that it actually is my hair ... we usually have a good laugh ... and they end up asking me for my methods to help restore their hair.

Many of my clients (both genders) are concerned about their dry hair, and loss of hair, and usually blame it on 'old age'. Where in fact, in most cases, hair loss is the accumulation and result of years of poor treatment and over-washing. After a while it simply 'gives up' ... and can't grow well anymore due to lack of nutrients. It is like a plant ... if it grows in poor earth with no fertilizers and poor care, it will whither, but once supplied with nutrients, it will become restored again and will be able to multiply.

'REVERSED' HAIR CONDITIONING
that really works!

This is probably the most effective treatment to regenerate your hair ... <u>with great results!</u>

- Put about 2 tablespoons of <u>good</u> conditioner (or more, depending on the length and thickness of your hair) into a cup, add a little water, to make it less thick ... so it can absorb well.
- Apply the mixture to your **UNWASHED, DRY HAIR.**
- Rub it into the scalp, make sure all your hair is saturated. This takes about 1 to 2 minutes ... and rinse.
- Now shampoo ... and then rinse, rinse, rinse – so no shampoo residue is left in your hair and scalp.
- As a last step, add a small amount of conditioner into your hand and rub through your hair ... and rinse.
- Do not comb your hair while it is still wet! It breaks easily when wet.
- Let it air-dry and wait for it to be nearly dry, then bend down, so your hair will hang toward the floor ... and gently brush it with a wide-spaced brush. This is not only a good exercise for your back, but will also brings blood to your head ... good for hair and skin.

HOME-MADE CONDITIONERS

Here are treatments which helped keep the hair of the Empress (and mine) in excellent condition. When I was young, my hair was quite thin ... it was nourished with the following conditioners.

These simple and inexpensive ingredients are usually found in your home.

RAW EGG CONDITIONER (on dry hair)

◆ one raw egg yolk – passed through a sieve for smoothness.
◆ massage into dry hair and scalp before shampooing.
◆ cover with shower cap or plastic bag ... let soak and absorb for about 5 minutes.
◆ rinse thoroughly
◆ shampoo ... and rinse **thoroughly.**

◆ **for a final rinse:** mix one cup of cider vinegar with 2 cups water, pour over hair, catch solution in a bowl and repeat   -
(the odor will fade within a few minutes, and in addition leaves the hair lustrous).

.

OLIVE OIL CONDITIONER or JOJOBA OIL
(on dry hair)

- warm oil to a comfortable temperature
- massage into dry hair and scalp
- cover with shower cap or plastic bag
- leave on for about 5 minutes
- rinse thoroughly
- shampoo as usual and **rinse thoroughly**

Here is another simple **HAIR RINSE:**

- boil about 4 cups of water, pour over 4 tea bags of CHAMOMILE and let steep.
- pour over hair, catching solution in a bowl to repeat 2 to 3 times.
- you can use this also for a face wash ... at the same time!
- Chamomile will add golden highlights to blond hair ... or, as an alternative, you can use fresh lemon juice with water ... which also adds golden highlights.

I usually plan my hair-treatment time on my 'day off' – so I can incorporate the drying-time with my projects or ... relaxing time.

I let my hair dry by air, without the aid of a blower, this way it will have a chance to regain its natural luster. I only use a dryer if it is absolutely necessary ... in case of cold weather.

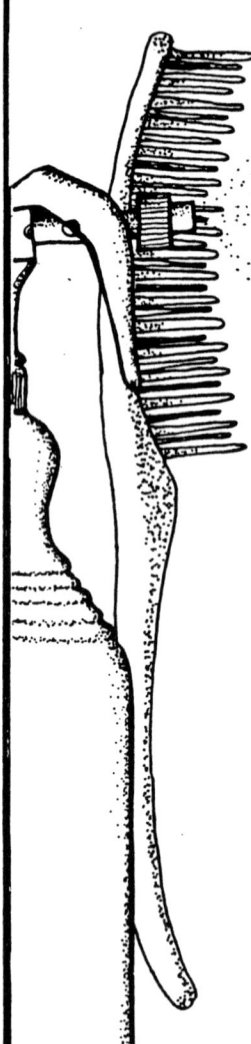

I brush my hair with a wide-spaced scalp brush which is an excellent multi-tool! You can also use it, while taking a bath to stimulate your skin and especially the bottom of your feet!

Once your hair has had a 'vacation' from hot blowers it will change it's appearance and becomes more manageable ... and all the time you spent restoring it, will be well worth it.

If you need help in keeping your hair in 'place' – use a *plant sprayer* filled with Aloe Vera juice or watered down Aloe Vera gel. It will not dry as quickly as commercial sprays ... but it will keep your hair in place without the additional chemicals.

THE STIMULATING FACE SCRUB

It was always an adventure for me when my grandmother came to visit from the United States. She would unpack a variety of surprises and beauty treatments which were then compared to my mother's finds of European origin.

No matter in which country we resided, neighbors would come and visit and over a cup of tea asked questions about new treatents from America. I realized at an early age the importance of looking one's best (for **oneself**) was of great interest to ladies from all continents ... and I knew then that I was destined to eventually follow in the same footsteps.

One of my grandmother's as well as my mother's favorite rejuvenation methods was exfoliating the face, neck and body on a daily basis.

One of their favorite concoctions was mixing a few drops of honey with finely ground almonds into a basic cream – making a somewhat rough consistency. At times, my grandmother used mashed potatoes, but always added finely ground almonds, which she seemed to use for nearly all her beauty treatments.

I tried both of her recipes and still use them with some variation. However, I have found two commercially available 'scrubs' which I use on a regular basis with great results, especially if I don't find the time to prepare my own mixtures. After all, when I heard about exfoliation for the first time about 68 years ago ... products of that nature were not as available as they are now.

So as you can see, I was taught to scrub my skin ... from face to toes at an early age. At that time I used a very rough washcloth and then eventually added exfoliate granules.

On the other hand, since I came to live in the U.S.A., I heard and read that the face should be washed gently in order not to damage the skin ... the exact opposite of what I was brought up with. But what about face-lifts and other aggressive and expensive methods of facial rejuvenation? They certainly are not 'gentle' ... and usually only last a few years, in addition to making the individual look somewhat 'different' from one procedure to another, depending on the results of the physician's artistic ability.

While all this different information may seem confusing, I did make my own decision about my skin, based on my own experiences. Since I don't believe in face lifts (unless absolutely necessary) I make sure that my skin remains clear of dead skin cells which accumulate on a daily basis and hamper the skin from breathing properly.

Since the skin is constantly in the process of renewing itself, it is very beneficial to help it along by removing the old cells with stimulating granules. Sloughing off dead, flaky, hardened cell build-up helps remove that drawn, tired, dry look. Just a few treatments will make your skin look better and feel smoother. You will also have better results if you don't use makeup foundation – most can dry out your skin and clog the pores – and not to forget – it can stain your clothes.

I exfoliate every day, and think of it as a 'mini-micro-peel' - making sure that my skin can breath properly, assisting the skin's natural process of rejuvenation. And most importantly - in addition – supply the system with the best nutrients possible.

I think of dead skin cells like the dead leaves on the lawn which will prevent most of the watering from reaching the soil and new grass, by absorbing most of the moisture. When one rakes the dead leaves away ... the new grass will be able to get all the needed moisture to regenerate. <u>This is just like our skin - remove the dead cells and the new skin will be able to breath, absorb and maintain moisture in order to regenerate.</u>

For me, the exfoliating treatment is most comfortable when relaxing in a bath - this way I can also scrub my elbows and toes – to keep them smooth. I scrub my face every evening (or morning), alternating with light to rougher textures. I never use soap for my face, there is no need – the scrub takes care of cleansing and stimulating.

Here is all I do:
I spread a light layer of exfoliation scrub over my wet face, neck and shoulders, and rub with wet fingers, in rolling circulating motion. I do not use pads ... the fingers are sensitive and let me know if I am over-doing it, or, if I am too close to my eyes ... then I rinse with tepid water. I DO NOT DRY MY SKIN WITH A TOWEL - I just wring out a washcloth and wipe my skin moist ... then I apply my chosen moisture cream over the still damp face.

Here are the formulas I was brought up with. You probably have most of the ingredients as part of your supplies in your kitchen!

To make:
Mix ingredients in a small bowl until they form a meal-like mixture.

ALMOND-HONEY SCRUB:
- ¼ teaspoon HONEY, or
- ½ tablespoon MOISTURIZING CREAM of your choice, or, ALOE VERA GEL
- 2 tablespoons finely ground ALMONDS (a blender will do this perfectly)
- mix thoroughly and apply.

MASHED POTATOE-ALMOND SCRUB:
- ½ cup mashed cooked POTATOES
- 2 tablespoons finely ground ALMONDS
- mix thoroughly and apply

CORNMEAL – MASHED POTATOE SCRUB:
- 2 tablespoon fine CORNMEAL
- ½ cup mashed cooked POTATOES
- mix thoroughly and apply

Don't forget to soften and beautify your feet! You can use all of these treatments to help remove the rough spots and calluses and get your feet to look their best and get them ready for your favorite sandals.

SMOKING – A DEADLY, POISONOUS HABIT

You can use all the beauty tricks in the world ... and you might even succeed for a while – but if you smoke, you should seriously consider ending this life-snuffing habit ... which does not only affect you ... but others around you!

Smoking leaves the skin looking dead and opens up the pores, giving out a repugnant odor from your skin, breath and clothes. You won't be aware that you are constantly walking around in your own polluted 'cloud'! Even the use of breath fresheners will not mask the tell-tale odor ... there simply is no escape from the negative side effects.

The effect smoking has on health in general is very serious. Many of my clients suffer from a variety of throat conditions and other health issues ... mostly due to the habit of smoking.

Many degenerative diseases and illnesses are directly linked to cigarette smoking, such as lung cancer, respiratory ailments, chronic bronchitis, heart disease ... just to mention a few. The use of smokeless chewing tobacco can result in cancer of the mouth, tongue, lip, throat, larynx ... and other related health problems.

My eyes were opened to the reality of cigarette addiction during World War II. Since tobacco and cigarette papers were not available, smokers invented a variety of concoctions, of which _strawberry leaves rolled in newspaper_ was the most popular. One might think that strawberry leaves would be fragrant ... but it must have been the addition of newspaper that created a horrible odor, which I am unable to describe!

I know that was one of the major reasons why I never developed the desire for smoking ... aside from being told that it was 'unlady-like' and would contaminate my lungs, stain my fingers and eventually make my skin ugly. The latter was probably the strongest reason ... vanity!

Smokers have told me that licorice sticks and cinnamon bark help during the times when they are trying to quit.

NOTES ...

CHAPTER FOUR

PMS & MENOPAUSE

GOOD NEWS
HORMONE STIMULATION THERAPY
WHAT TO WEAR WHEN TRYING TO REDUCE
THE LANGUAGE OF THE BODY
INTESTINAL CLEANSING
SOY AND THE THYROID
AIR CONDITIONING AND ITS DETRIMENTS

PMS & MENOPAUSE

I have never resorted to hormone therapy. Instead, I took special care to continue to eat a low-stress, pH-balanced diet and also increased some of my supplements ... in particular I supported my **ADRENAL GLANDS** so they would be able to supply me with the needed hormones. I refer to this as:
HST ...HORMONE STIMULATION THERAPY!

It seems that women are conditioned from an early age to believe that they must suffer physical pain and mental distress during these years ... with the possibility of even losing their femininity. The customary symptoms of menopause including 'PMS' can be blamed on the accumulation of years of stress, habitual bad nutrition, depriving the body of necessary nutrients ... resulting in undermining the whole system.

This is why it is so important to start EARLY IN LIFE with proper supplements ... that are personalized according to one's deficiency – so the body is supported during various stages of stress, whether it is from over-work, lack of sleep, PMS, menopause ... or simply feeling overwhelmed.

GOOD NEWS!

When the ovaries have stopped producing estrogen (one of the essential hormones that give women their feminine characteristics), nature has set up a **BACK-UP SYSTEM,** the
ADRENAL GLANDS!
Among the key hormones produced by the adrenal glands, are ADRENALINE, ESTROGEN, CORTISOL, TESTOSTERONE, PREGNENOLONE, DHEA ... all essential to maintain good physical and mental health. If the adrenal glands are depleted, they are unable to produce the necessary hormones. The healthier the adrenals, the less one will suffer common general, **PMS** and **menopausal** symptoms. Overworked adrenal glands are easy to detect ... the symptoms usually start with nervousness, lack of concentration, forgetfulness, edginess ... and **FATIGUE,** which often leads to **DEPRESSION.** After all, how can one feel joy, if one is tired and stressed? Most people notice a decline in their energy between noon and late afternoon, regardless of age and gender. At that point, life seems a total bore!
I like to make a point of always including BOTH genders in the subject of stress because the initials PMS are often used in a rather derogatory way, in reference to women when they

are under a certain condition. However, when a man acts stressed ... the simple conclusion is that he had a 'hard day'!

I believe that the term PMS should not be used at all, and should be replace with:
AES ... ADRENAL EXHAUSTION SYMPTOM.
<u>This of course would apply to both genders!</u>
This certainly would remove the negative aspect of the original term.

Many women approach menopause in a state of emotional and nutritional depletion which affects optimal adrenal function. In particular, women who had children must take special care to eat healthful foods with supplements in order to help regenerate their depleted system ... and this will also prepare them for the years to come.

You can see again how very important it is to have a system which is **supported according to IT'S NEEDS,** and which is not required to overwork some bodily functions on a constant basis ... as in menopause. This also explains why those who support their body at an early age have less negative symptoms ... compared to those who neglect to assist the first signs of deficiencies.

When adrenal glands are depleted, one is much more likely to suffer from fatigue and menopausal symptoms.

I try to think of the adrenal glands as the body's primary **SHOCK ABSORBERS.** These two little grape-size glands, that are on top of the kidneys, are designed to produce hormones that allow us to respond to the conditions in our daily life with enthusiasm and energy ... which in my mind is **JOY! And, the adrenal glands, when in top shape, support the immune system!** However, if the intensity and the frequency of the stresses in life become too great ... <u>the adrenal glands will become depleted</u> ... like a car without gas! And you are much more likely to suffer from fatigue, over-all health problems and menopausal symptoms.

If one is hypoglycemic, the symptoms are often more pronounced. Stress puts a burden on the adrenal glands, causing them to over-work. In that case, the adrenal glands produce smaller amounts (if any at all) of the hormones that are needed to help reduce the side effects of menopause.

Again, the ease of transition into menopause depends upon the strength of the adrenal glands and the state of your general health.

So, don't wait until menopausal symptoms overwhelm you. Support your system and the adrenals as soon as possible and in every way possible!

**This is the time to do something about supporting your health
DON'T WAIT UNTIL OTHER, MORE SERIOUS SYMPTOMS SHOW UP!**

Several of my clients have said that their doctors have taken them off HRT based on the latest reports.

So, instead of
"HRT" ... HORMONE REPLACEMENT THERAPY
why not try
"HST" ... HORMONE STIMULATION THERAPY

A NOTE for those who are taking **PREMARIN:**
PREgnant **MAR**e ur**IN**e ...

I would like you to be aware that it is made of a **pregnant mare's urine** ... if you doubt this, just put a drop of water on a tablet of the Premarin ... and smell it!
I will not go into the horrible details of the extreme pain the mare has to go through ... but I feel it is important to at least let you know ... **THAT IT DOES!**

You have a choice to take alternative measures!

HORMONE STIMULATION THERAPY ...
THE ADRENAL GLANDS AND VITAMIN B-5

Over forty years ago I started to seriously choose supplements which would aid the various functions of my body ... I was about 35 years at the time. I am certainly glad I started then, even though supplements where not as obtainable as they are now.

In addition to my basic vitamin and mineral combination, I add **PANTOTHENIC ACID,** which is also referred to as **B-5,** or, the 'anti-gray-hair factor'' and the 'stress vitamin'.
I am often referred to as 'Panto-Benita' due to my strong belief in it and the great results I achieve for myself, and my clients.

According to scientific research, <u>B-5 is essential for the production of the adrenal hormones</u> ... **it helps revive them!**
The **ADRENAL GLANDS** (cortex and medulla) are two triangular Endocrine Ductless Glands situated on top of the kidneys.

As I mentioned previously, some of the hormones produced and secreted by healthy adrenal glands are: **estrogen, cortisol, adrenalin, testosterone, pregnenolone, and DHEA.**

However, as with any supplement, whether vitamins, minerals, herbs, amino acids, etc., you have to take caution and know your limits ... especially if medications are also involved.

As an example in case of B-5, If you take more than your body requires, B-5 might increase the heart rate and blood pressure! And ... consumption of caffeine causes release of excessive adrenaline heading to future depletion of adrenaline! A good reason to stop coffee all together.

To find out if you need additional B-5, a good measure to go by is your energy level between noon and afternoon, around four p.m. If you find you are sluggish and can hardly keep your eyes open ... **then you know you are in need of supporting your adrenals glands.** As I mentioned before, I have supplemented with B-5 for over 40 years, and believe me ... it has helped in so many ways ...noticeably, my energy level. When I did not add B-5, for whatever reason, I felt a decline in my energy and in my concentration, within 2 to 3 days.

If you decide to add B-5 to your vitamins, here are my suggestions ... it requires your close attention!

If you work during the day, you would have your breakfast in the morning, around 7a.m. to 9 a.m. ... and that is the best time to take vitamins. They have to be taken early in the day, unless you work at night ... it takes them a certain amount of time to be absorbed. If you take them without food, you will most probably feel ill. If you take them at night, and it is the amount your body needs ... you most probably will have trouble going to sleep.

If you work at night, take your vitamins at your dinner time ... or the meal before work. This way they will help assist you during your work time ... if you take the right amount.

Everyone requires a different dosage of any vitamin, and most definitely with B-5. The amount one needs, depends on the level of depletion of the adrenal glands.

Always start low ... start with 250 mg <u>with your breakfast, and your multi-vitamins</u>. If you only take B-5, without a multi-complex, you will be depleting your reserve of other vitamins. B-5, <u>needs</u> it's <u>family</u> of B's to be absorbed properly ... if it is on it's own, it will leach the vitamins it needs from your body.

If you don't feel more energy in the afternoon, you know you can increase B-5 **the next morning** by an additional 250mg.

The afternoon will indicate to you if you took the right amount needed by your adrenal glands.

When I was going through menopause, in my 50's, I required 1500mg daily, and for the last few years I reduced it to 1000mg. This might seem a lot in comparison to other vitamins, but one has to go by what the body requires ... everyone has different reactions. This is why it is important to know the pros and cons of supplements.

The quantity is important. Remember, taking more than your body requires will give you a feeling of having had too much coffee to drink, or, even being somewhat 'edgy' ... this is not the feeling you want! So listen to your body if you should decide to supplement with B-5.

On the other hand, taking less than your body needs, will not increase your energy or feeling of wellness. Sometimes when ... let's say, 1000mg is not enough, and 1250mg is too much ... it might help to get the right amount, by breaking one 250 mg tablet in half, to reach what you are comfortable with.

WHAT TO WEAR WHEN TRYING TO REDUCE

For over twenty years I designed and manu-
factured clothing and accessories for the
"Missy" market. I created a timeless look
which was simple and could be worn by
most any one.

During my fashion shows, I had the opportunity to meet many of my customers and
realized that most of them wanted to hide
their weight ... instead of changing their diet
to help trim their lines. Two specific styles re-
peatedly sold out, regardless of what was
currently in vogue. One was a simple, clas-
sic dress, that looked good on any age and
any figure – and had the effect of visually
slimming the wearer. The other was a two-
piece, easy-fitting pantsuit, which looked
good any time. The order and sales of these
styles never failed to confirm that most
women have a concern for their weight ...
and are always looking for something to
conceal it. This is one of the reasons which
gave me the idea of compiling this book
...to help women direct their energies into
improving themselves, rather than wasting
energy by searching for the sort of garment
which would hide bulges ... the direct result
of bad habits!

When in the process of losing weight it is important to wear simple lines that don't reveal what you are trying to lose ... or hide. During this time especially, one should take special care to look one's BEST ... so one does not become discouraged and give up before one sees actual results. <u>Enjoy what you wear ... even if you are only going to the market!</u>

Your aim should be - never having to apologize for the way you look! You alone are responsible for your appearance and the impression you create. The feeling of looking your best will increase with every pound you shed ... **all it takes is for YOU to start**.
<u>But, my advice is never talk about it!</u> It will be such a disappointment if no one notices. Let your friends notice your changes for themselves. This way you will KNOW it's an obvious improvement and <u>that</u> will encourage you to continue with even more determination.

**It is so much more rewarding
to look better as we grow older, rather
than ONLY to have enjoyed
good looks in our youth!**

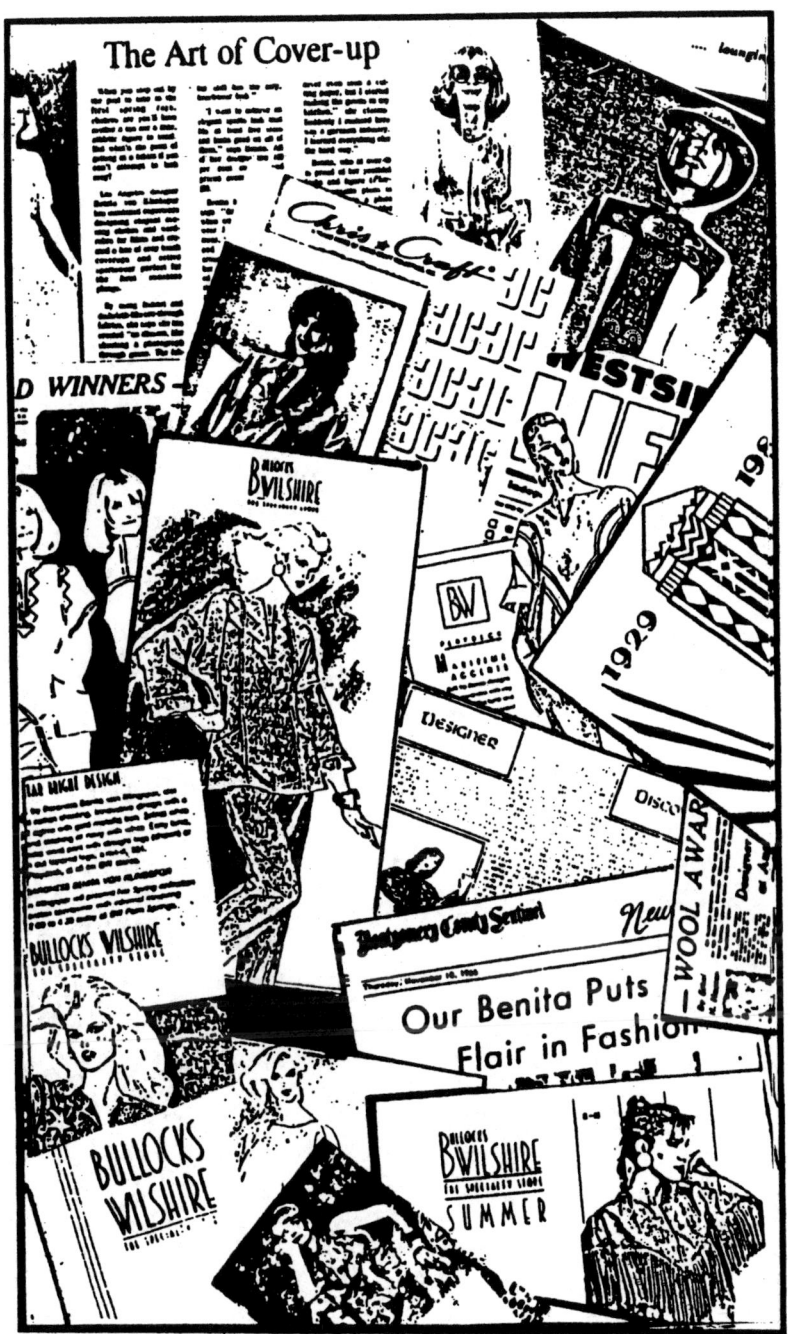

The Art of Cover-up

WINNERS

Our Benita Puts
Flair in Fashion

BULLOCKS WILSHIRE

BWILSHIRE
SUMMER

THE LANGUAGE OF THE BODY

When I studied 'preventive medicine' or, also referred to as 'alternative healing' - the most interesting topic to me was 'symptom-atology', which I think of as *the language of the body* ... understanding the connection between nutrition and disease. The body gives us indications through discomfort, which helps us ... in most cases ... to identify the source of the aches and pains, which usually means that something needs our attention.

Since we are born without an instruction manual ... we should learn what the body is telling us. Once we understand, we will be able to help eliminate what might be in the developing stages ... **no matter how unim-portant the signal might be or seem at the time.** On the other hand, if we don't listen, we will get to know the **LANGUAGE OF DISEASE**. It is truly best to catch everything in the very beginning stages. Just like a small snag in clothing ... or the strange sound in a car or equipment, or a plant which looks frail. If I neglect to take care of the first warning sign, more difficult indications will make themselves known.

In a way, the body is like a message center. Every part of the body has its own signal in order to communicate when we are neglectful. I believe in reacting right away by taking care of the problem at hand and support regeneration by supplying my system with what it is lacking, or, eliminate the foods or over-use of supplements, which could also be the cause of the problem.

If I neglect to react to the signals, I will have to experience the consequences.

If you are taking medication, or, you have a medical condition, it is best you check with your physician before taking any additional supplements. Your symptoms might be due to side effects of the medication and by taking additional supplements, you might interfere with the medication or cause yourself harm.

Here are a few of the major complaints (indications) from my clients and what can help them in most cases.

Bruising ... trauma to the skin ... blood leaks out of the capillary walls and collects underneath the skin.

Bioflavonoids with a high amount of **Rutin** (1000mg) have the ability to increase the strength of the capillary walls and to regulate their permeability.

It takes about 2 to 3 months to strengthen and repair the capillary walls ... depending on the deterioration.

Burns ... superficial burns from ironing or a hot stove or even a sunburn ... try this:
slice a raw potato very thin, so you can practically see through the slice ... and apply to the burn. Or, if your hand is burned ... submerge your hand into a bowl filled with grated raw potato ... you will feel the soothing effect within minutes.

Constipation ...is often due to a diet lacking in raw, green vegetables ... chlorophyll contains magnesium, important for the digestive and elimination process and other bodily functions. You might add additional magnesium to your supplements, however, if you take too much ... you will experience diarrhea.

Diarrhea ... if the digestive system is unable to assimilate fats, diarrhea is often the result. Also, check your supplements ... if various combinations include magnesium, you might be exceeding the amount your body needs ... and, you will experience diarrhea.

Mucous ... sniffles, post-nasal-drip and general sinus problems ... often occur when the body is highly acid from too many starchy carbohydrates and/or protein and colas. The body is in the process of eliminating the excess acidity. In many cases, people think they have continued colds or flu ... and continue to take cold medication, where in fact, they should try to eliminate or cut way down on the amounts of starches and proteins in their diet.

Slippery Elm bark extract can speed up the removal of mucous ... it is safe and also benefits the stomach lining and the intestinal wall.

Fluid retention ... this is a condition in which excess fluid is retained by the body ... swelling is most often seen (and felt) in the hands, the rings on your fingers feel too tight, the feet, the ankles swell and the eyes are puffy. This could be due to an unhealthy diet ... too much salt intake.

Dandelion root is very helpful in eliminating water retention. I consider it the best herbal diuretic; it contains potassium and other electrolytes ... and helps digestion.

If you are on medication, or have medical problems, it is best to consult your physician.

Leg cramps - appear more frequently in the elderly, often due to magnesium deficiency, or lack of circulation.

Headaches ... with too many starchy carbohydrates, sugars, sodas or diet drinks you are inviting all sorts of trouble ... hypoglycemia (low blood sugar) is one ... which eventually could develop into diabetes. Headaches are one of the symptoms. Change your portions of food to more green vegetables (they are low in carbohydrates) and supplement with 400mcg GTF chromium ... glucose tolerance factor.

If you are experiencing any of these symptoms, and you are on medication, don't take any additional supplements until you have discussed your discomforts with your physician ... who is familiar with alternative healing.

INTESTINAL CLEANSING ...THE COLON POTION

Think of it as "Spring Cleaning" ... it is very helpful to clean the intestinal walls from all the accumulated toxic debris three to four times a year.

If you are not 'regular' ... try eating more fresh, green vegetables ... they contain fiber and magnesium, essential for colon health. Make sure you are drinking enough water, half your body weight in ounces is a good measure to go by. Also one of the side effects of taking medication can be constipation.

There are many products available, but I always go for the simplest program. Here is my colon potion:
♦ Place one heaping teaspoon of **PSYLLIUM SEED HUSK** and one teaspoon of **BENTONITE POWDER** into a mug.
♦ Add your choice of liquid ... and mix.
If you add water, it will taste sort of like 'cardboard' ... if you add juice, the mixture will take on the taste of the selected juice.
♦ Stir thoroughly and drink **IMMEDIATELY**! If the phone rings ... let it ring! Don't answer it, if you do, the mixture will be solid by the time you return to your 'potion'.

If the mixture gets 'thick' while drinking, add more liquid ... don't let it get too thick ... to the point of gagging, otherwise you surely will not try this healthful procedure again!
♦Make sure you drink more water than usual.

Take this 'colon potion' once in the morning and once at bedtime for about three to four weeks. If this is your first time ... start with just three to four days ... and repeat after one week. Once you are 'seasoned' you can do this routine for a month. I believe it is always best when one introduces the body to new procedures to start with smaller portions ... crawl before you walk!

I am often asked if this potion will cause diarrhea or other digestive reactions. All it does, is clean your intestinal walls and simply gives your stool a better form. Remember to drink more water than usual.

While I am on the subject of cleansing ... listen to your body and go the bathroom when necessary. Do not ignore the urge, if you do, over time, this habit may cause the ability to eliminate more difficult, in addition to creating other health problems.

SOY AND THE THYROID

Years ago, when soy powder became popular, I decided to add it to my smoothies ... in spite of the warnings I read about soy, I thought they were exaggerated.

However, after about four weeks of using soy powder, my thyroid blood test (TSH, T3,T4) indicated an alarming increase in my TSH level, which means my hypothyroid condition (low thyroid) was getting worse. Then I knew that the articles I read about soy were true: **"soy inhibits the production of thyroxin!"** Five weeks after discontinuing soy, my TSH test indicated that my thyroid improved greatly, and eventually I was able to bring it to a normal level.

Several of my clients, who also have a low thyroid condition, mentioned that their medication had to be increased since they included soy in their diet. However, once they removed soy from their diet ... their thyroid tests improved considerably.

Dr. Mike Fitzpatrick, (New Zealand) has extensively researched the impact of soy consumption on thyroid function ... and that soy can have a substantial impact on anyone with hypothyroidism. Over-consumption of soy products, like: tofu, miso, tempeh, soy milk, soy drinks, various soy supplements, can cause enlargement of the thyroid and can suppress thyroid function.

If you do not have a low thyroid condition, soy might not affect you. However, the only way you can really know if your thyroid is functioning correctly is by having a TSH, T3 and T4 blood test.

Since I have a low thyroid, I also add extra vitamin B-2 to my multi-vitamin. This by the way, also helps when one experiences on occasion 'watery eyes' – 100 to 200mg per day.
In addition, since cruciferous vegetables, like cauliflower, broccoli, cabbage, also inhibit the production of thyroxin, try to add other finely-cut vegetables, to your meals like: asparagus, bamboo shoots, bell peppers, celery, cucumbers, daikon, green beans, parsley, radishes, zucchini. If you never had a Greek salad ... this might be just the time to try one.

Also, since the liver is unable to convert beta-carotene into vitamin "A" in the case of a low thyroid ... it might be a good idea to add 10,000 IU of dry vitamin "A" to your supplements.

AIR CONITIONING AND ITS DETRIMENTS

If I am in an air-conditioned area for only a short while ... I know that I will most probably experience earache, sore throat, swollen glands, and possibly a neck and shoulder ache. I know that I am not coming down with a cold or flu ... but these symptoms are the direct results of being exposed to a draft or cold air on a hot day. Believe me, I try anything to stay away from such situations.

When I lived in Hawaii, I found that the contrast of the humidity and the air-conditioned stores caused everyone I knew discomfort resulting in flu-like symptoms ... the body will eventually succumb to the contrast of overly air-conditioned surroundings to out-door conditions, which is a shock to the system.

If you are close to a draft either created by an open door or window, fan, or air-conditioner ... try to divert it or stay out of the path of the stream of air. This applies also to gym areas, when one wants to cool down after a workout. Also, many of my clients, who experience hot flashes and night sweats, try to create an environment of cool air brushing over their skin. After a short while they often feel the results of a flu-like condition.

In addition, air-conditioned areas have an extremely drying affect on the skin.

If you want to aid your dry skin, try this simple, but useful aid:

If you have a small plant-sprayer or a refillable purse-sized sprayer, you could convert it into a mister for your face.

Clean the sprayer thoroughly, so that no

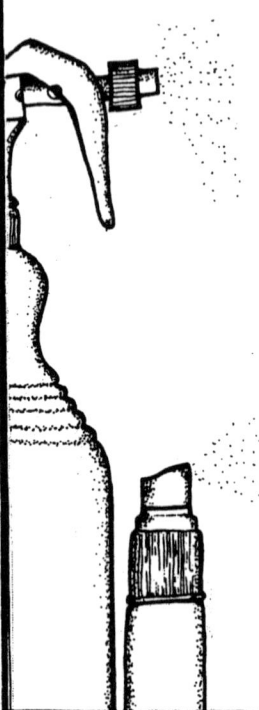

chemical residue remains in the bottle or spray channel. Fill with purified water and spray a light mist over your face and neck several times a day. It has a cooling affect, helps keep the skin moist, and is a great pick-up on a hot day. It feels especially good while driving in a hot car.

There are a great variety of over the counter sprays available.
Make sure you select the one with the <u>finest mist.</u>

CHAPTER FIVE

YOUR RESTFUL HAVEN

TIME TO START A PROJECT
IMPORTANT LESSONS I LEARNED
CREATE A RELAXING AREA ... YOUR HAVEN
THE LOW-COST MINI-HEALTH SPA
THE MINI-GYM
GIVE YOUR CLOSET A FACE-LIFT
FIRST AID SUPPLIES

TIME TO START A PROJECT

Projects are very important to me. I always feel that I have to create something ... it gives me a great feeling of satisfaction and is the best therapy I can think of, whether I draw, sew, or simply change my living areas.

I was brought up quite isolated from other children – except for attending school. My mother was concerned that I might pick up bad manners ...so, strict standards of behavior and protocol brought discipline into my life at an early age. This consequently taught me self-discipline ... a valuable asset in facing the trials of adult living.

I was tutored in drawing and painting, and was taught by my mother and governess how to sew, knit, crochet and embroider, and how to entertain myself with projects. In "those" days, dolls were popular ... and they became the silent victims of my sewing creations. By the time I was five I had no trouble finding something to do, which I truly enjoyed, and to this day, I still find pleasure in all these arts ... which turned into hobbies ... and eventually my chosen profession.

Drawing and art gave me the opportunity to accept a position as art director at Hughes

Research Laboratories in Malibu, California.

Sewing, on the other hand ... directed me to establish my own design and manufacturing company. For over 20 years, I created garments and accessories for women and children ... won the 'wool award' – a prestigious award in the garment industry. So, my little 'silent victims' who were forced to wear my creations when I was taught how to sew ... certainly served a purpose in my life.

The guidance I received in nutrition at an early age created an interest to pursue this subject on a higher level in order to maintain a healthy system ... and eventually help others as well.

So as you can see ... a project is a good thing. All the instructions, guidelines and discipline of years ago did pay off and still fill me with the joy of being able to create whatever I feel like doing ... stick with it, and do it to the best of my ability.

I follow certain guidelines, which help me with my project at hand ... they might be helpful to you as well.

Here they are:

♦ Don't feel you have to create something, **JUST to do something.** If it is not what you truly want, you will lose interest.

♦ **"See"** your item first, see it in use, and most of all 'enjoy' thinking about it.

♦ When you make your final decision, **refine each step** in detail in your mind. You can do this while relaxing ... taking a bath ... a walk.

♦ Make a **rough sketch**, which only you need to understand, and note what you will need in materials.

♦ Have your **tools in good shape** and keep any small hand tools in attractive containers; let them become a part of your environment.

♦ **Pick colors YOU like.**

♦ Create your **own style** - not what you think someone expects of you.

♦ **Start with the easiest part** ... the rest will follow and unfold itself to you.

♦ **Complete each step to the BEST OF YOUR ABILITY, add improvements as you progress.**

♦ If you come to a point of confusion, **STOP** ... go on to another part of the project ... or have a nutritious snack ... do stretching exercises. Absence of a few minutes will do wonders!

♦Don't work until you are totally exhausted, it will leave you with a negative impression on your mind and it will become difficult to talk yourself into completing your idea.

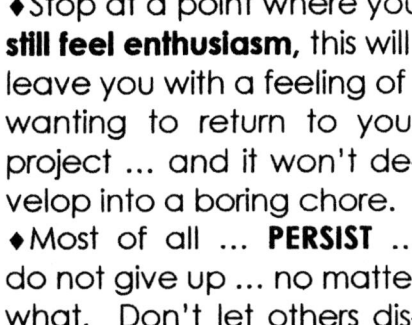

♦Stop at a point where you **still feel enthusiasm,** this will leave you with a feeling of wanting to return to your project ... and it won't develop into a boring chore.

♦Most of all ... **PERSIST** ... do not give up ... no matter what. Don't let others discourage or influence you.

♦**BEST YET** ... keep it to yourself, until all is done! Then you can 'unveil' your creation.

♦When you are done for the day, re-organize your tools, so they are ready for your next endeavor. You will start looking forward to those quiet, well-spent moments working on your project!

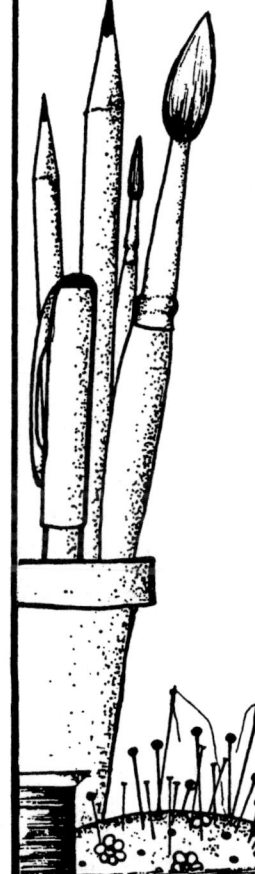

If you decide to start a project, don't invest much time for the first idea. Why not check the unused jewelry that you might have forgotten and stashed away ... disassemble the various pieces and create a new look!

If you feel like sewing ... and have not done so for quite some time, or never ... start with a simple item, which will not require much time. A small purse to hold your essentials is always useful ... even for a gift.

The easiest one to create, is one that does not have to be lined! Get a few yards of medium to strong ribbon – about 2 inches wide ... gros grain is always a good choice, because it is stiff and easy to work with, and it comes in many colors. Decide if the bag should be closed, either with 'velcro' or zipper or snaps, or simply a large flap. You can make a simple design or add beads.

Figure out what size you want your bag (front, back and flap) ... cut the ribbon to that length. If you want a bag six inches wide, then cut three lengths, over lap the edges slightly and sew on top of the ribbons to hold the edges together. Once you have all three lengths sewn together, you can create the final shape.

Forgotten, tucked
away necklaces
become
new treasures
and   ...

old clothes
and scarves
turn into
usable things,
like purses ...
or whatever
your imagination
can create.

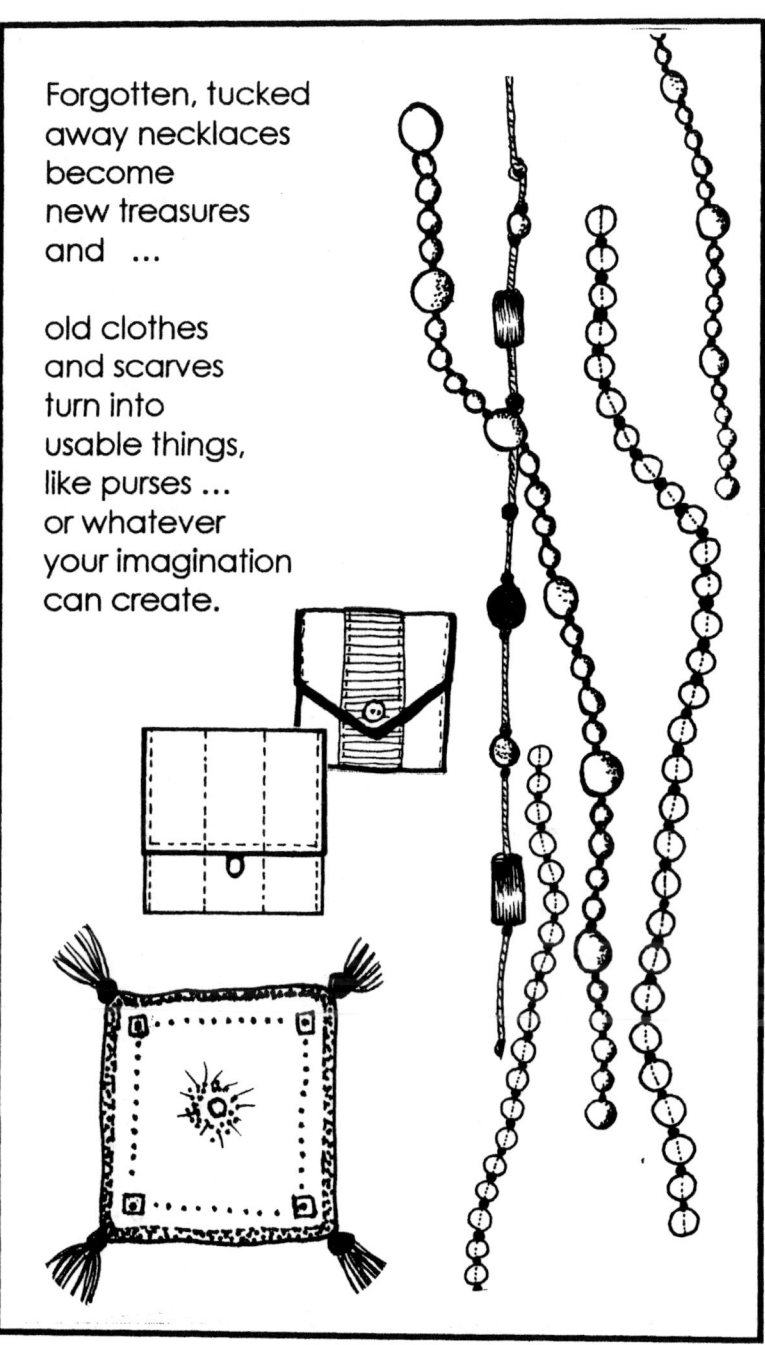

IMPORTANT LESSONS I LEARNED

Persistence will reveal the results of my dreams and will help me get there in spite of so-called failures. Most of all however, every project, no matter how insignificant, I do with enthusiasm and to the very best of my ability, so that I can be satisfied with the results.

During WWII, I remember large, beautifully designed posters with slogans in gothic print which were posted in schools, air raid shelters, even throughout the debris of bombed-out buildings ... they stated:
"ARBEIT MACHT FREI" - *"FREUDE DURCH ARBEIT"* and *"KRAFT DURCH FREUDE"* ...which mean: **"WORK GIVES FREEDOM"** - **"JOY THROUGH WORK"** and **"STRENGTH THROUGH JOY"**. These statements, when seen on a daily basis, can't help but penetrate the mind - they certainly remained in mine!

To this day, goals and projects are important to me. However, they must be crystal clear, otherwise they will eventually fizzle out. I try to set a goal high enough to demand my best and to develop a burning desire and passion to complete it. Without a goal, days just seem to 'float' by, leaving me with a feeling of dissatisfaction.

Eventually I also learned that failures give me an opportunity to learn something new on the way to reaching my goal ... it may delay me but it won't keep me from getting there. Mistakes often directed me on a different path, with new and additional ideas which usually added greatly to my overall project. However, if I allow myself to dwell on the problems, they simply under-mine my enthusiasm to press on ... and the project usually develops into a boring chore.

It seems, mistakes are just diversions which give additional options to create the very best ... that is, if one stops and listens!

Clients often tell me that their goal is to retire and to relax after years of working. However often, months later, they find themselves searching for something worthwhile to do, regardless of age. So, don't be fooled if you are toying with the idea of retiring ... unless you have something very special in mind to fill your free hours.

PERSISTENCE IS AN ESSENTIAL ELEMENT

EVERY GOAL IS WORTH THE EFFORT IT REQUIRES

CREATE A RELAXING AREA ... YOUR HAVEN!

I find pleasure in rearranging my living area for two reasons: to make it the ultimate in comfort ... and to be visually pleasing.

If you do not have a relaxing area where you can be by yourself, find a secluded and quiet 'away-from-it-all' place in your home were you feel comfortable. Create an area exclusively devoted to your mental well-being, <u>no matter how small this peaceful spot may be.</u> Should you feel there is not such a space available, perhaps that should tell you it is time to discard some superfluous possessions which are only gathering dust.

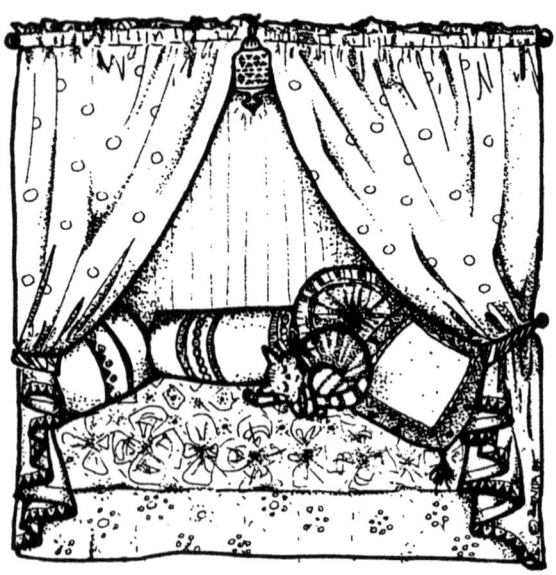

Some of the no longer wanted or not used items could be 're-cycled' into active use by someone who really needs and wants them. This will also give you the inner joy of having contributed to someone else's well-being, and will give you the required space for your "comfort space".

You really require very little to create this new comfort station for yourself ... a few colorful pillows, a blanket, a soft rug, candles in a safe spot, a plant ... and YOU! And, if you are lucky enough to be owned by a cat, you can really learn what relaxing is all about.

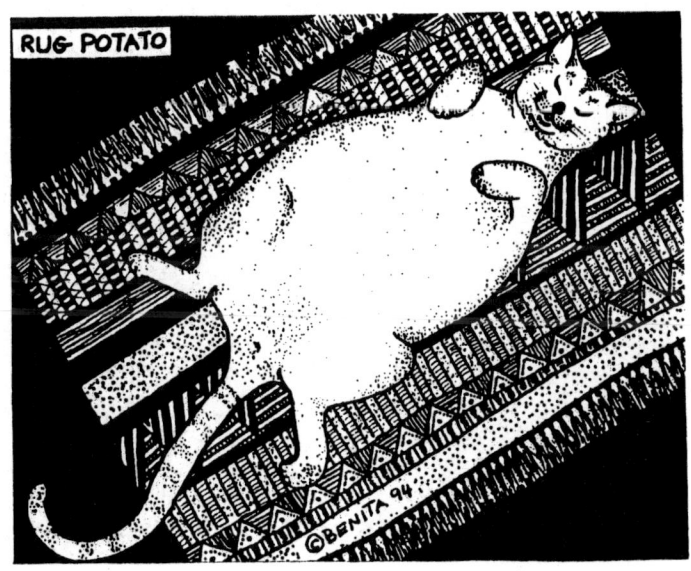

RUG POTATO

THE LOW-COST MINI HEALTH-SPA

The more pleasant an atmosphere you can create in your personal mini health-spa, the more it will become associated in your mind as a haven of rest for the ultimate in physical relaxation and comfort, where you can make yourself look and feel good.

Make these moments a regular habit, they will help relax you ... so important for your total well being. Conversely, the result of not taking time out for your personal needs will leave you feeling dissatisfied and drained.

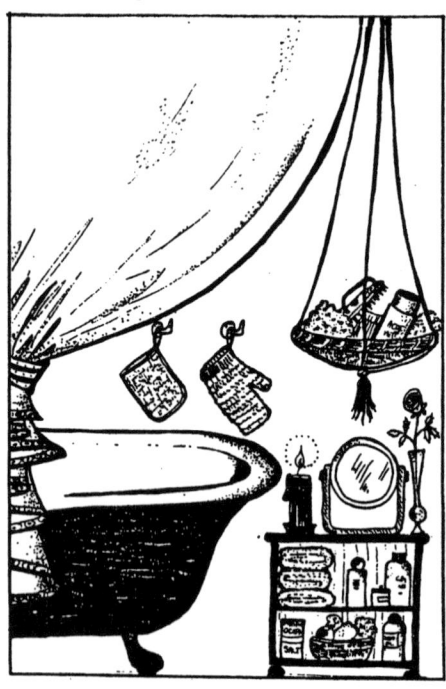

To me, a bath is one of the most enjoyable pleasures in life. I have always taken great care in decorating my bathrooms - my spa. I usually add light-weight drapes, reaching to the ceiling to the already existing sliding doors ... they help keep the air warm, which makes the whole bathing experience a more comfortable and lasting pleasure.

Throughout the war years, and long after the war, before normal order was established, my dreams were of lounging in a steaming bath, filled to the brim with warm water, un-interrupted by fear of bombs and the sound of explosions. Fantasizing about the pleasures of bathing, became a form of wishful thinking.

In those years, no one dared to risk being caught in the bath. Eventually, bathing had become a thing of the past anyway, not only due to utilities being shut off, but also due to destroyed pipes and the contamination of water.

Collecting rainwater during the summer and snow during the winter, helped immensely - just to have water for washing. The winter months added more complications ...towels were not able to dry due to the freezing weather and consequently left moisture on the skin, which resulted in frostbite ... a most painful condition. There was nothing we could do to help alleviate the pain, except wrap our swollen (to the point of bursting) hands and feet in thick layers of cloth to keep the skin from being exposed to the freezing atmosphere. Shoes, gloves and mittens did not fit over the bandages. Rings had to be cut off due to the extreme and sudden swelling of the fingers.

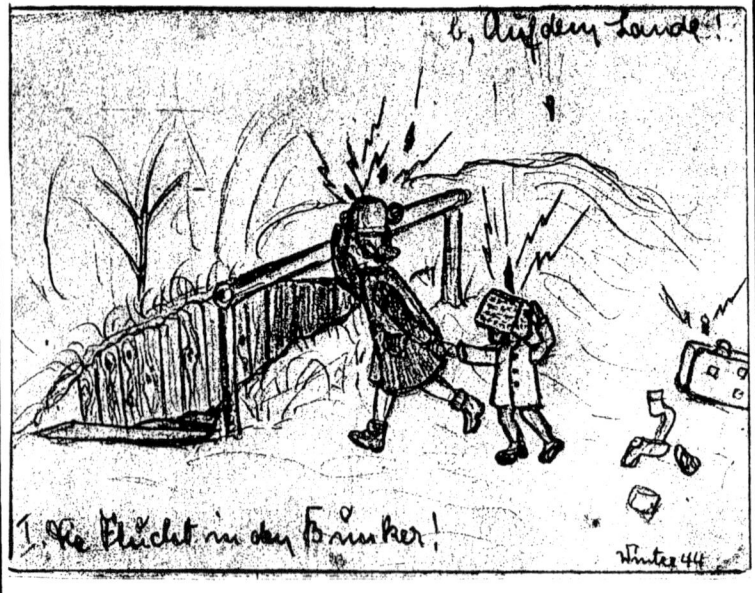

This is one of my drawings (WWII/1944).
You can see, that taking a bath was the last thing on our mind, when one had to run for shelter from bombs and shrapnel at any given moment.
Here we are escaping to a trench in a bombed-out area
Pots and sturdy bags were used to protect
our heads from shrapnel and debris.

To this day, decades later, I still take great pleasure in the simple joys of being able to lounge in water, the fulfillment of my dreams from WWII. I know I will never be able to take these moments for granted. I am sure you can understand why.

So, when I take a bath, I take advantage of these moments by making them into a real beauty treat, not just a way to get clean. Soft music ... candles ... and all my beauty tools handy ... the scene is set.

After relaxing for a while, I start to exfoliate my face, neck and shoulders. Then scrub the hands, arms and especially the elbows, legs, and a thorough scrub to the bottom of the feet and toes, finishing with the whole body. I always keep in mind, to massage toward the heart. This treatment is an exercise in itself, just to reach all the areas, especially the back! However, for that, I have a wonderful tool, which can be used wet or dry – the "RIFFI" back-scrubber.

As a finale, a thorough rinse with an extended shower head, an essential addition for every bathroom. It removes all suds, feels wonderful ... and makes cleaning the bathtub very easy.

No matter how out-dated the bathroom might be, small changes and additions could give it a new look and transform it into your new mini-health-spa. A few wall hooks will hold your rejuvenating tools necessary for your forth-coming program, and if you have the space, add shelves to hold your towels, lotion, bath salts, mirror, and not to forget ... a candle, in a safe place.

Here are some of my most favorite beauty tools:

♦A **rough washcloth,** I usually purchase a bartop-cleaning cloth because of its strong fibers, and a **rough towel** - both of these are needed for additional exfoliation.

♦**'RIFFI-brand' mitten** and **back-scrubber,** I can't imagine bathing without either of these great-feeling tools ... the back-scrubber reaches every part of your back without struggling ... it can be used dry or wet ... and it is great for the bottom of your feet, by simply 'slinging' it under your feet. Once you have tried them, you will wonder how you ever managed without them. They are particularly helpful in cases of poor circulation.

♦**Exfoliating granules** for face and neck, are most important. I like to keep two types on hand. One by **'TAUT'** which has delicate granules, and one by **'derma-E'** ... with stronger, more condensed granules. Both give me the results I love to feel and see.

◆A chemical-free **moisturizers** by **'ALEXANDER AVERY'** – either the Almond, or the Dream cream. Both of them feel great ... the cream is dense, therefore it is important to make sure the face is WET ... it makes it easier to apply.

Of course you can add lots of other items... but I like to make everything simple and only use what really works.

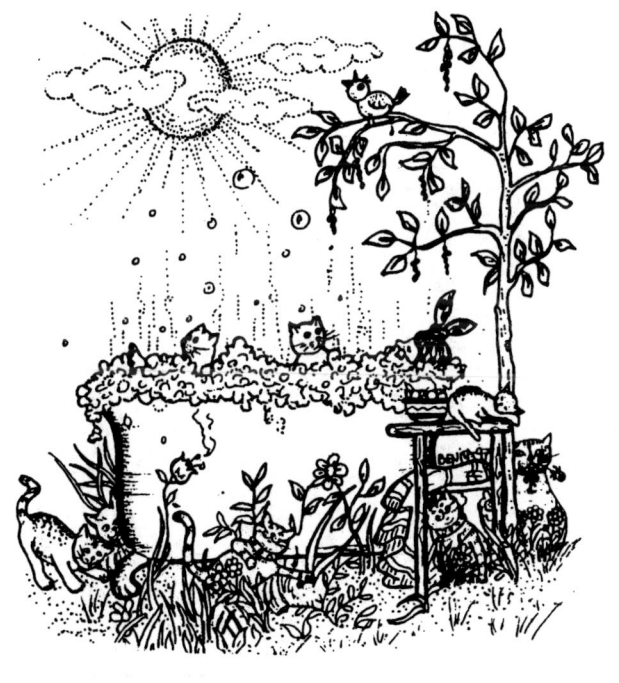

THE MINI-GYM

I have difficulty keeping my walls blank. They all seem to have a purpose ... either with wonderful pictures or lots of plants. But I usually find a small area, maybe 5 feet wide for a mini-gym ... a constant reminder!

If you are serious about starting an exercise routine, you might convert a small area into a 'mini-gym'.

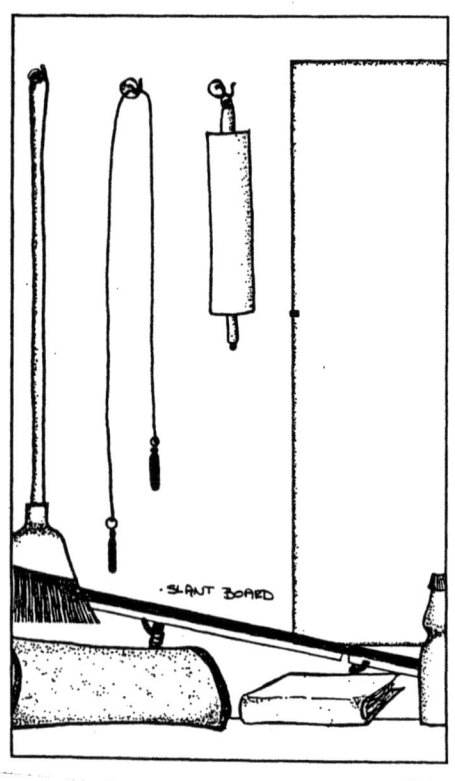

Create a visible area to help promote your new life-style which will make it easier for you, instead of stashing your exercise tools in a closet... 'out of sight - out of mind'! You need only a few basic items to 'stock' your home gym.

♦ A full-length **MIRROR** (which will be also helpful when you dress)
♦ An exercise mat or a large towel.
♦ A **BROOM** or **'POSTURE WAND'** which I mentioned in "Don't create your own 'Dowager's Hump" (Chapter 1).
♦ Two empty **BLEACH BOTTLES** (they will weight 3 lbs each when filled with sand)
♦ A **JUMPROPE**
♦ A **ROLLING PIN** ...for thighs and general workout
♦ A **SLANT BOARD** if the space allows
♦ And if you wish and want to spend the money ... you can invest in some colorful **WEIGHTS** ... that will help tone you ... and add color to your décor.
♦ A few ornamental **HOOKS** to hold your tools.

THE STAGE IS SET for your 'performance' and the 'rave' results! ... You could have a gym party with your friends ...   ending it with delicious healthy smoothies ... or veggies, or fruit ... a simple and delicious feast.

GIVE YOUR CLOSET A FACE-LIFT

When I decide what to wear, I want to be able to find it right away ... and in ready-to-wear condition. Searching for whatever I want is a waste of time ... and certainly could be most frustrating.

So, when you open the door to your closet, do you feel uninspired? Are your clothes too tightly packed, hard to find, unshapely and do they make you feel unattractive?

Why not re-do your closet! Re-organize and generate more space. Make it a JEWEL BOX, with all the necessary accessories on display and close at hand.

Don't keep your closet as a storage center with hidden piles, old boxes and faded, outmoded clothes that are not YOU anymore.

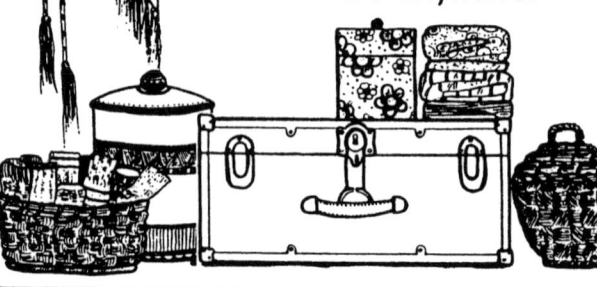

Make it a workable place that aids in your all-over beauty program ... your very own BOUTIQUE!

To generate space, the following steps always help me in deciding what to keep and what to discard. Try them, they might be helpful to you too.

I usually make three piles of all my accumulated items:

1. The splendid things:

Those are the clothes and accessories I know look good on me and that I love wearing. I make sure that they fit, are clean and are ready-to-go. Then they get a special place in the closet on good hangers. Good hangers are important, they help in keeping the clothes hanging properly. I certainly would not use wire hangers ... they ruin the clothes and also I think they look ugly.

2. The undecided things:

They might become functional again if the fabric and colors are some of my favorites. That is, it I have the time to recycle them into a new look, bags or pillows. I often hang on to some items for sentimental reasons. However, in most cases, they simply remain forgotten in their designated box ... 'out of sight, out of mind'. So I usually give them to someone who would be able to use them.

3. The ugly things:

If they do not look good on me ... then **out with them**! They can become a rag, only if the fabric is suitable. I do not want to keep items that are unattractive, uncomfortable and not repairable. But mostly, I don't want to keep anything that I would have to apologize for, or have to hide when wearing it.

If you really want a total change for your closet and have the time to spare – cover the walls with fabric, paper or paint them. Add a few ornamental hooks for your bags, scarves, and belts; baskets or fun boxes to hold your socks, scarves, and the items to be altered. A colorful sack is good to hold your to-be-washed items ... and not to forget ... a full-length mirror is important to make sure that all looks good.

Your imagination is the only limit!

FIRST AID SUPPLIES

Always be prepared ... it is a good idea to keep a variety of first-aid supplies and popular herbs on hand.

I listed only a few benefits from the herbs. Here is the list of helpful items:

- **Band-aids**
- Two-inch square **gauze**
- **ACE bandage**
- **Safety pins**
- **Colloidal Silver salve**, essential for mosquito bites, rashes, scrapes, hives, itching.
- **Colloidal Silver 500 ppm liquid**, useful for sore gums, sensitive teeth, sore throat ... but not to be used on a regular basis.
- **Goldenseal root** powder, very helpful in case of mouth sores, general sore gums.
- **Oil of clove**, helps in case of tooth ache, it numbs the gum area for about 20 minutes.
- **Slippery Elm** extract, extremely helpful in removing mucous when taken every hour, also soothes stomach and intestinal lining.
- **Aloe Vera** concentrate, helpful with digestive problems and intestinal discomfort.
- **Charcoal** capsules, helpful in case of food poisoning and gas.
- **Acidophilus**, helps regenerate good intestinal bacteria.

◆ **Ginger Root** capsules, helps to prevent motion sickness, improves blood circulation.

◆ **Dandelion Root**, a potassium rich herb, it is a superior natural diuretic, helps reduce stiffness in the joints. (Not to be taken by those without a gall bladder).

◆ **Peppermint Tea**, is a gastric stimulant, it is primarily used to alleviate stomach and intestinal problems.

◆ **Hawthorne Berries** in capsules or liquid, is used primarily as a cardiac tonic, it is effective in regulating rapid or feeble heart beat, helps in lowering blood pressure, relieves restlessness and insomnia.

◆ **Fennel Seed**, helps in weight reduction by curbing the appetite and alleviating hunger pains ... therefore in Austria it is referred to as the "seed of obesity" – it helps reduce the formation and build-up of uric acid tissue.

◆ **Cayenne** is a healing spice and does not corrode the stomach lining as black pepper does. It also helps prevent frostbite ... it was most helpful in keeping us warm during the cold winter months in WWII. We often sprinkled a small dusting of powder into socks and mittens to keep us warm and to prevent frostbite.

It is best to consult with your physician. Some of the herbs might interfere with your medication.

CHAPTER SIX

BEING A VEGETARIAN

BEING A VEGETARIAN
DID YOU KNOW?
GREEN FOODS
PROPER pH BALANCE
THE DIFFERENCE BETWEEN TEAS
HOW TO BREW A PERFECT CUP OF TEA

BEING A VEGETARIAN

According to my mother ... as an infant, I never liked fish, chicken or meat, regardless of how it was disguised on my plate. Even though I was not aware of 'what' the substance was, I remember disliking the texture, odor and feeling I got from just looking at it.

And then one day, the truth was revealed. I shall never forget grade school in Prague, Czechoslovakia ... the day the teacher pointed to a large painting of little pigs in a meadow ... told us about them ... and then explained that they were killed to be eaten, by humans. It was then when I realized with horror, that the 'stuff' on my plate – which I never cared for ... was the remains of a slaughtered animal! I could not comprehend how one could eat what once had been a living creature.

After that day, I looked at everything on my plate with great suspicion ... and only felt comfortable eating what was green ... or a vegetable or fruit I could identify. Please understand that I lived a very sheltered life and never knew about unpleasant things until World War II ... when EVERYTHING in life as I knew it in Czechoslovakia and other countries changed over night.

Shortly after that, we left Czechoslovakia due to the political turmoil. My mother and I were traveling through Germany in order to be able to board the last ship to America ... when what we tried to escape from in Europe became a reality ... the borders were closed ... it was the beginning of World War II.

Oddly enough, this major occurrence did not only change my life in many ways ... but it also was the beginning of my foundation as an accepted 'vegetarian' – and I was no longer thought of as a child that was a fussy eater. My mother, a British subject, had far too many serious problems to take care of at that time in Germany ... which was at war with her country. So, my choice of foods was no longer a point of concern for her and certainly became less important.

I realized then, that I was not so odd after all. Quite a few people were 'vegetarians' ... even though I did not understand why one had to make such an official distinction between eating or not eating animals. However, the day when ration cards were distributed ... I realized that mine, in addition to being a different color ... replaced animal parts with butter and cheese.

You can't imagine the feeling of freedom I experienced ... being able to eat foods that I truly liked. However, that was a short lived victory ... food became very scarce due to the bombing episodes. I must say though, that being a vegetarian made life easier for me during those years ... in comparison to others, who thought they needed meat, etc., and were more structured in their need for certain foods. I was quite content with just having vegetables, and simply eating them in their raw state ... which, by the way, everyone eventually had to resort to anyway, due to the lack of electricity and gas.

I must add, that the schools were very informative about what to eat. One particular day always comes to my mind, and I also mentioned it in one of my other books ...
"IS THERE ANYTHING LEFT FOR ME TO EAT?".
One of the teachers brought a bouquet of daisies into the classroom and each one of us received one, which we had to place in our inkwell on the desk. We had to draw the daisy from various sides, and leave them there until the next day. When we returned in the morning all the daisies had turned a light blue color ... and that was our introduction to:
   'HOW FOODS BECOME A PART OF US'.

When I moved to the U.S.A., vegetarianism was not yet really recognized. It seemed as though I had to start all over to convince others that my choice of eating was healthy.

I feel, too much emphasis is placed on protein ... here, vegetarians are told to eat beans and rice to get the protein they need. So, in most cases, they overdo this. In fact, most of the 'vegetarians' who come to me for counseling have extreme fatigue, low blood sugar, candida, allergies, and mainly sinus problems.

The cause of these symptoms is due to over-consumption of starchy carbohydrates and far too few fresh, raw vegetables. High amounts of starchy carbohydrates make the body highly acid. However, when reversing these proportions and placing more emphasis on raw vegetables, this helps in making the body more alkaline ... and, can make a great difference in anyone's health.

Those who have read my book regarding pH-balance, know that starchy foods and protein are highly acid-forming, causing an unhealthy acid pH. An imbalanced pH can start with congestion, sinus problems, skin problems, joint pain, digestive complaints, weight gain and can lead to the progression of most, if not all, degenerative diseases.

I am often asked if I am tired and bored of vegetarian food. That is a simple question to answer ... because how can I be tired of food I enjoy? It is the simplest way of eating and so easy to digest. In most cases people eat more or less what I eat ... just in different proportions.

A. They might select:
about **three cups of pasta or rice (starchy carbs) with**
one cup green vegetables (non-starchy carbs),
which makes this a highly acid-forming meal and high in starch.

B. I would select:
about **three cups of vegetables (non starchy carbs)** ...and only **one cup of pea or lentil soup (starchy carbs)**
which makes this a highly alkaline-forming meal and low in starch.

The food is the same, the only difference is the proportion ...
"A" is high in starch and highly acid forming
"B" is low in starch and high in alkaline nutrients.

I am also often asked how I get protein. This too is simple to answer. When I have one cup of pea soup ... I get about 18-19 grams of protein .... and by adding garbanzos to my vegetable salad, I get more protein ... in addition, everything that comes out of the earth has a small amount of protein as well. So, as you can see ... there is enough protein. This way of eating has kept me healthy throughout the decades ... and now, at near-75, my blood tests and bone scans indicate no problems.

However, by comparison, eating large amounts of protein could be a problem ... it leaches calcium from the bones, it is hard on the kidneys and it is highly acid forming, which can open the door to a variety of health problems.

The majority of people I counsel have allergies. On top of the list are congestion, sniffles, sinus problems and post-nasal-drip, to name just a few.
And guess what ... in most cases these symptoms can be easily eliminated, simply by eating less starchy carbohydrates, less animal protein ... and more fresh, raw vegetables and fruit!

There is one more thing I would like to add about being a vegetarian. Many of my clients call themselves vegetarians, even though they eat fish ... they have been told by other sources that it is all right to include fish in their diet. However, a vegetarian never eats anything that has to be killed ... and a fish certainly does not jump around for joy when being caught. So, whether, a creature has no legs, two legs or four legs ... it is not included in a vegetarian diet.

A 'vegan', on the other hand, does not eat anything from a live or dead creature ... this includes dairy and honey.

I must admit ... about forty years ago, every once in a while I indulged in lobster ... I love the taste. But ever since (40 years ago) I saw an educational film about lobsters and other sea creatures ... I had to abstain from the delicious taste of lobster. I observed how the hundreds of lobsters were walking close in a long chain on the bottom of the ocean ... and then were swept up by fisher-men to be served as delicacies. The next stage of course is ... being thrown alive into boiling water or hacked in half, etc. This was too much for me and I was unable to make another excuse on behalf of my desires. Believe me, this was a test ... but I stuck to it.

DID YOU KNOW....?

Did you know that in two pounds of charcoal-broiled steak there is as much benzopyrene (cancer causing agent) as in 600 cigarettes?

People who eat meat have a higher risk of getting cancer because of the carcino-genic preservatives added to meat like nitrites, nitrates, and other preservatives which are added to mask the green discol-oration that occurs as the meat ages. These preservatives are injected into the animal so they will circulate throughout it's body, often causing the animal's death before being slaughtered.

Urea and uric acid, both nitrogen com-pounds, are the most prominent wastes collected in the body from a meat diet. Beefsteak contains approximately 15 grams of uric acid per pound. The kidneys have to work much harder to eliminate toxic com-pounds from a meat diet, than that of a vegetarian diet.

Raw meat is in a state of continual decay. It will contaminate everything it comes into contact with, including the cook's hands.

Did you know that when you cook the fat in meat at high temperatures, as is most frequently done to sear it and seal in the juices, methycholantrene is formed, another cancer-stimulating substance.

Did you also know that chickens often retain estrogen pellets ingested to promote growth and plumpness. If it affects chickens ... what about those who eat them!? Also, the antibiotic, tetracycline, added to the chicken's feed, has been linked to severe food poisoning.

When the body is younger it can handle the extra work of a meat diet without any outward signs of harm, but as the body ages the kidneys cannot work as efficiently.

The following is a list of complaints that can be directly linked to the over-consumption of meat, starches and dairy products: Sinusitis, congestion, hives, skin problems, impaired digestion, obesity, constipation, diarrhea, edema, gas and bloating, fatigue, allergies, headaches, depression, anger ... and the list goes on! These are just a few symptoms of an **OVER-ACID SYSTEM**!

GOOD NUTRITION, BASED ON pH BALANCE WILL HELP THE BODY PERFORM PROPERLY

GREEN FOODS

GREEN FOODS ... so important for all of us, are the major part of a vegetarian diet.
Green foods are rich in chlorophyll, a collector of the sun's energy. Chlorophyll is the green pigment of plants required for photosynthesis ... and is sometimes referred to as "plant food". This substance is similar to the hemoglobin of our red blood cells, though rather than containing iron at the cell center, as found in human blood ... chlorophyll contains magnesium.
Chlorophyll's benefits are numerous. It is highly alkaline, is an anti-inflammatory, aids digestion, speeds wound healing, and due to it's magnesium content, aids elimination.

Green foods are often called 'superfoods' ... because of their high nutrient content. Here is a closer look at some of the green foods:

ALFALFA ... This member of the pea family is the most common source of commercial chlorophyll.

BARLEY GRASS ... derived from the young grass of planted barley.

BLUE-GREEN ALGAE ... this superfood is found

in freshwater lakes and reproduces rapidly. Upper Klamath Lake in southern Oregon is the only place in the world where large quantities are available in the wild. Blue-green algae is 65 percent protein and, because the cell wall is soft, it is easy to digest.

CHLORELLA ...this single celled, fresh-water algae is believe to have existed on earth for about 2.5 billion years. Chlorella is rich in protein, it contains 19 of the 22 amino acids and, with 12% chlorophyll, is the highest source of this nutrient. Studies show that it <u>stimulates white blood cell production.</u>

SPIRULINA ... another blue-green algae. It was used by the Aztec Indians as a daily food and trade item. It grows in warm alkaline or salty water ... and contains 65% protein. In fact, one acre of spirulina yields 20 times more protein than an acre of soybeans.

WHEAT GRASS ... this superfood is sprouted from wheat berries. Wheatgrass contains 17 amino acids and is a rich source of vitamin C, calcium, iron, magnesium, germanium and zinc.

CHLOROPHYLL IS LIQUID SUNSHINE!

PROPER pH BALANCE

One of the first questions I usually ask my clients is about their diet. Most of the time they try to assure me that their meals are well-balanced ... however, in most cases, their consumption of starchy carbohydrates is high, as well as their protein intake, and their fresh vegetables and fruits are at a very low minimum.

When starchy carbohydrates and protein are the majority of a diet ... the body will eventually suffer from over-acidity, resulting in sniffles, sinus and throat problems, ear-aches and skin problems. If these symptoms are ignored, the body will succumb to more serious conditions.

In my book: "IS THERE ANYTHING LEFT FOR ME TO EAT" ... I wrote in detail about how modern diets cause an unhealthy acid pH.
In fact, diet appears to be the major influence in maintaining appropriate pH levels throughout the body.

All biochemical functions are severely compromised if oxygen supplies are decreased to living tissues. <u>A diet high in fresh green vegetables will help supply oxygen to living tissues which will increase the alkaline state of the body.</u>

Ideal proportions between acid- and alkaline-forming foods are around 20% to 80%.
I prefer to estimate in quarters:
25% acid-forming and
75% alkaline-forming foods.

A **3:1 ratio** will provide you with a properly balanced pH diet:

3 CUPS fresh, raw VEGETABLES
ALKALINE-forming
(or, slightly steamed)
with
1 CUP GRAINS or LEGUMES
ACID-forming

Percentages within each nutrient often vary due to different harvest times, maturity of the plants and soil conditions.

♦**All GREEN VEGETABLES** are alkaline-forming
♦**NO-STARCH AND LOW-STARCH VEGETABLES**
and potatoes are alkaline-forming
♦**acid-forming vegetables:** cress, rhubarb, corn and all winter squash
♦Most **FRUITS** are alkaline forming, except: blueberries, plums prunes, and cranberries.
♦**All GRAINS** are acid-forming, except: Millet
♦**All ANIMAL PROTEIN** is acid forming: including meat and all meat products, poultry, fish, shellfish ... and DAIRY.

Using foods alone can take a long time to correct an overly acid condition, unless it is minor. There are a variety of pH-balance supplements available to speed up and help correct this condition.

Many of my clients are concerned about the skin problems of their children, including acne.

These conditions are also most of the time the direct result of eating a diet high in refined starchy and sugary foods ... not only "junk" foods ... but also breads, cereals, and general starchy carbohydrates ... and sodas.

Articles often state that *"primitive populations are virtually free from skin problems"*.
I hardly consider the countries I lived in as *"primitive"*! However, what we had in common with these populations, was eating foods that where wholesome and supported health. Of course in those days we were fortunate not to be subjected to enticing and misleading commercials. Some teachers actually went to the extent to demonstrate that the inner part of white bread or buns should be removed ... and that it was only useful to help clean stained walls!

In addition to creating an acid condition, too many starchy carbohydrates and sugars will result in the release of excess insulin, causing <u>low levels of blood sugar</u>. Eventually the body is unable to keep up with the repeated demand for the release of insulin, and will result in <u>high level of sugar in the blood</u> ...**DIABETES!**

The only solution is to eliminate refined items and minimize the amount of starchy foods. Increase the selection of fresh green and other vegetables and add fruit to the diet.

A LOW GLYCEMIC DIET, which refers to foods that turn into sugar SLOWLY – (good mix of fresh vegetables, fruits, and some whole grains) keeps insulin levels low, preventing glucose resistance and fat storage ... and may reduce the risk of diabetes and other conditions.

The presentation of the food is important. Serving chunks of vegetables, especially in salads is neither attractive nor pleasant to eat. The smaller one cuts, chops, grates, or slices vegetables, the more their individual juices will intermingle and create an additional flavor. Since most people do not chew their food long enough, finely cut vegetables are more pleasant to chew and consequently easier to digest.

THE DIFFERENCE BETWEEN TEAS ...
WHITE – GREEN – OOLONG – BLACK

Tea ... hot or cold, white, green or black, is the world's most popular beverage, after water.

Since I get quite a few questions about the various teas, I thought the following information might be of interest to you.

Tea leaves (Camellia Sinensis) are classified as **white, green, oolong or black.** The color is the result of the chemical changes that occur to the leaves when they are given time to oxidize or ferment before drying, and during the manufacturing process.

Tea leaves which have been dried without being given time for fermentation remain green in color ... **GREEN TEA.** When given a short time to ferment, become **OOLONG TEA,** and when given full time to ferment become **BLACK TEA.**

The final step is firing (pan-heating) which stops the fermentation process. This firing process causes the leaves to turn black and reduces the moisture content to 1%. The results of the fermentation process give teas their strong, rich, complex flavor.

So, basically, the eventual taste from tea depends on several points: ◆leaf-age before picking ◆soil in which the tea was grown ◆tea age ◆different drying procedures.

CHINA is the birthplace of tea and continues to produce more intricate varieties than any other country.

The most famous growing regions are: Keemun (<u>Black</u>), Dragonwell (<u>Green</u>), and Tikuan Yin (<u>Oolong</u>).

INDIA is the world's largest tea producer. The most famous growing regions are: Darjeeling, Assam and Nilgiri, producing nearly all <u>Black</u> <u>tea</u>.

JAPAN is a sizeable producer of almost exclusively <u>Green tea</u>. The famous teas are Sencha, Genmai Cha, Gyokuro.

TAIWAN, often called Formosa ... the bulk of the teas produced there, are: <u>Oolong</u>, which falls into three categories: dark, jade and almost-green tea.

SRI LANKA, often called Ceylon ... is the third largest producer of tea in the world. The three famous growing regions are Dimbula, Uva and Nuwara Elyia.

♦WHITE TEA ... are top leaves and buds. Hairs on the leaves give them a whitish cast thus the designation "White Tea" - which are steamed and then dried without being rolled and fired. The absence of withering, rolling and fermentation, leaves the appearance of the leaves essentially unaltered. The curled-up buds have a silver appearance and produce a very pale, gentle tea.

♦GREEN TEA leaves have been dried without being given time to ferment. Immediately after picking, the leaves are steamed or pan-fired, a process that destroys the enzymes that lead to fermentation. The leaves are then rolled and fired to complete the drying process. Green Teas have a subtle, more astringent flavor than Black Teas.

♦OOLONG TEA ... is processed like Black Tea but has a shorter withering and fermentation process to produce a tea with color and flavor somewhere between Black and Green Tea.

♦BLACK TEA ... the leaves are picked and then withered to reduce the moisture content ... they are then rolled or twisted and placed in a cool, humid room where they undergo a fermentation process (full-time, for 1 to 5 hours). Due to the difference in the fermentation process, a portion of the active compounds are destroyed in Black tea, but remain active in Green tea.

Tea is soothing and contains one third less caffeine than coffee or cola. It contains antioxidants, vitamins and minerals, and is a rare source of natural fluoride, which helps inhibit growth of the oral bacteria which are responsible for dental plaque.

Polyphenols are among the most talked about dietary ingredients these days. They are a class of phytochemicals found in <u>high concentration in tea, grapes, wine and a wide variety of fruit and vegetables</u> and have been associated with supporting the prevention of heart disease and cancer. Polyphenols are responsible for the bright colored pigments of many fruits and vegetables.

One of the more nutritionally important classes of polyphenols, the flavonoids, are widely distributed in plant foods and include:

Catechins (tea, grapes, wine)
Tannins (tea, nuts)
Anthocyanins (brightly colored vegetables and fruit)
Lignins (nuts, whole grain cereal)
Proanthocyanins (grapes, pine bark)
Isoflavones – genestein/daidzein (soybeans)
Quercetin (grapes, wine, onions)
Naringenin/Hesperidin (citrus fruit)

HOW TO BREW A PERFECT CUP OF TEA

Brewing is an art that is simple, but which also requires some care to do well.

- Use a preheated teapot.
- Boil the freshly drawn water.
- For **Black** and **Oolong teas**, bring fresh, cold water to a roaring boil and pour it over the tea leaves.
- For **White** and **Green teas**, use water that has just started to steam slightly. <u>White and green teas are destroyed with boiling water.</u>
- Add to your heated, empty teapot: one rounded teaspoon of tea leaves for each cup of water (one heaping teaspoon per mug).
- The amount of time to brew tea depends on the leaves being used and the individual's taste. Careful timing is essential.
- <u>General rules to follow are:</u>
The smaller the tea leaf, the less time required for brewing.
<u>Infuse Black tea for 3 to 5 minutes,</u>
<u>Green tea for 1 to 3 minutes,</u>
<u>White and Oolong tea for 2 to 5 minutes.</u>

If the tea turns out to be bitter or harsh, it is often a sign of over brewing.

NOTES ...

CHAPTER SEVEN

PHYSICAL
MAINTENANCE

DON'T HOLD YOUR BREATH
THE "5-WAY TWIST"
VARIOUS POSITIONS

DON'T HOLD YOUR BREATH!

Some type of exercise routine is essential for good health. It gives you form, keeps you limber, shaped, toned, sparks up the circulation, and promotes burning up those excess calories. If you think that a 'routine' is more beneficial in your lifestyle, set aside ten minutes each day and pick the exercise most suitable for you ... STAY WITH IT ... and make every move count!

Remember that **WE CREATE OUR FEATURES WITH OUR HABITUAL FACIAL EXPRESSIONS!** This also applies during exercise ... as you are in the process of 'making yourself over.' **RELAX YOUR FACE**, concentrate on each step of the exercise along with deep breathing and visualize your desired goals. **ENJOY** what you are thinking, and your face will 'follow suit' ... you are then creating a pleasant, relaxed expression.

BREATHING is as important as the exercise itself. Without sufficient oxygen, muscles can't function properly. Without oxygen, there is no life ... **DON'T HOLD YOUR BREATH!**

INHALE when you are at the greatest ease
with your position
EXHALE when you are making the most physical effort

THE "5-WAY TWIST"

In my teens, next to art, crafts and sewing, gymnastics was one of my most favorite activities. Aside from the daily calisthenics routine at school, the art of both gymnastics and calisthenics were perfected at the 'Jahn Turnverein' ... a leader of good form in physical fitness. That is when I received one of the highest awards for excellent routines on the parallel/horizontal bars and the horse. Of the many exercises I learned, to this day, the **"5-way twist"** routine is still my favorite one... mainly because I can take care of several areas at one time. It helps tone upper arms, diaphragm, waist, hips, and upper thighs. It combines toning with agility ... and with little effort produces profound results. I don't do them every day, only when I feel I need a change ... or my clothes feel snug – but, for visual results, it is best to make this a daily habit.

Following are a few basic tips to prepare for your general exercise routine:

♦ Make sure that you wear **loose clothing**, so air can circulate freely about your body. It is best to work out in open air ... or in front of an open window (not during heavy traffic time) ... and most important ... **NO DRAFT** to chill you. The body will react in some way or another when exposed to sudden change of temperature. **Drafts are often the unsuspected cause of muscle aches!**

♦ **Clear area** of objects. With some positions, you need more concentration ... subconscious fear of knocking something over or getting hurt in the process, only detracts from your intended benefits.

♦ **Wait** at least thirty minutes after eating to exercise.

♦ **To warm up** ... start with simple, slow, easy movements. **NEVER strain** yourself beyond your capacity!

♦ **Patience and practice** produce increased strength, endurance and confidence.

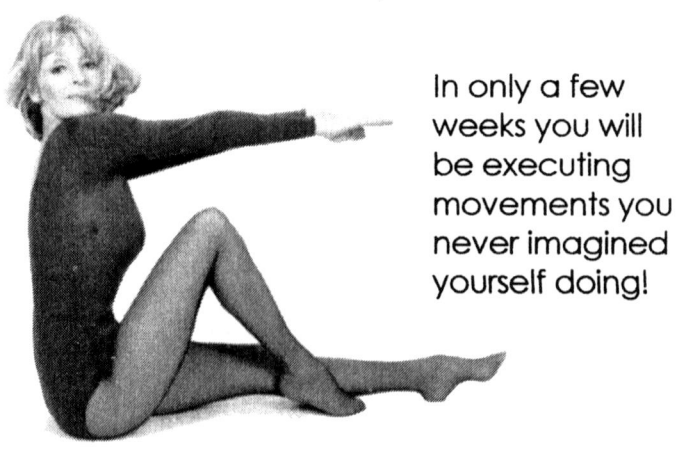

In only a few weeks you will be executing movements you never imagined yourself doing!

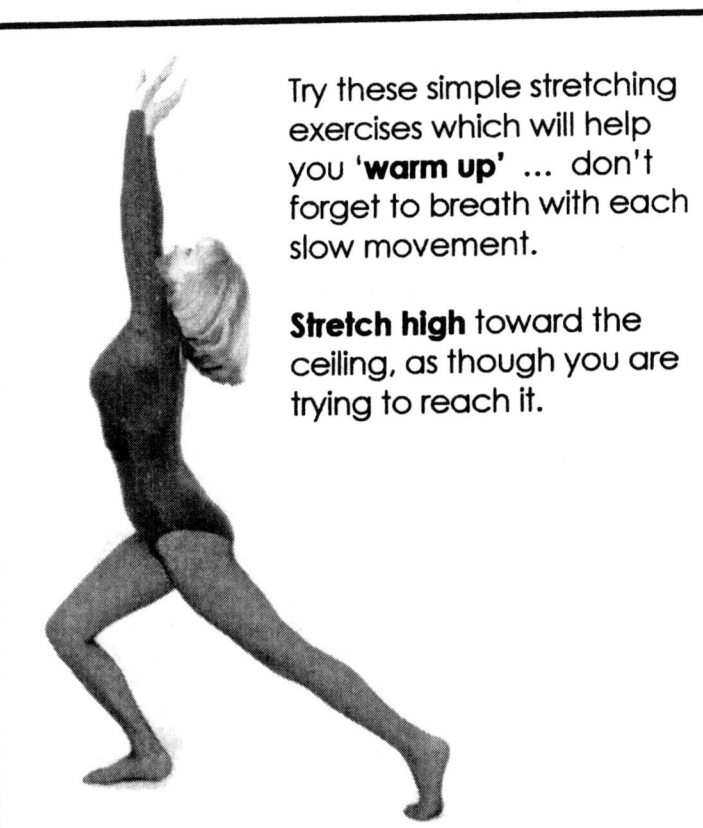

Try these simple stretching
exercises which will help
you **'warm up'** ... don't
forget to breath with each
slow movement.

Stretch high toward the
ceiling, as though you are
trying to reach it.

<u>INHALE</u>
when you are at the greatest ease
with your position
<u>EXHALE</u>
when you are making the most
physical effort

For the following **"5-way twist"**, you will need only a broomstick, or you can hold on to the base of the bed ... or, any solid object. Your body will have the tendency to move while you twist back and forth ... holding on to a solid object makes this routine easier. The photographs will show you how to position yourself. Make sure you **keep your upper arms parallel** to the broomstick (or solid furniture).

So, here goes :

♦ Lie flat on the floor
♦ Place the broomstick over-head on the floor, **holding on firmly** ... keeping your **elbows at a 90-degree angle.**
♦ Start by bringing your bent knees toward your chest ... **always maintain a tight grip in order to keep your balance ...**

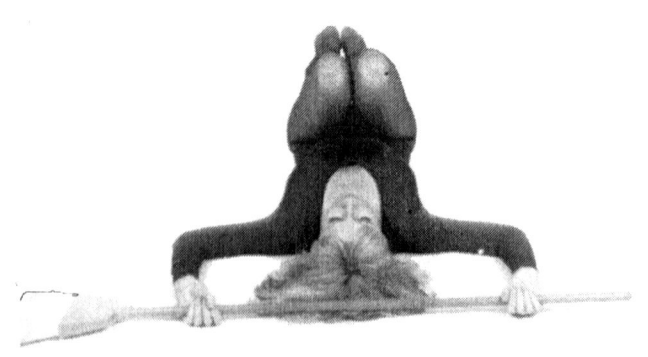

♦Once you are positioned with your **arms firmly holding the broomstick**, press shoulder and spine against the floor, while pressing knees together ... breathe in.

♦Now, while breathing out, **slowly twist the knees to the left side** ... try to touch the floor with your left knee ... press the upper spine to the floor. Take another breath.

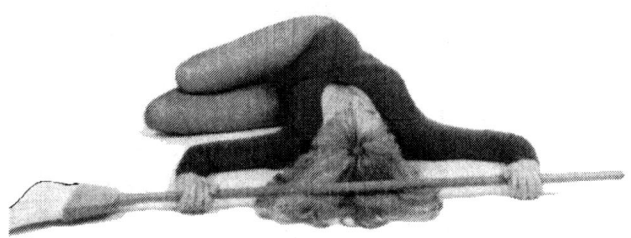

♦On the exhalation **slowly twist the knees to the right side.**
If at first you can't reach the floor with your knees, **DON'T PUSH**! You will become more agile as you practice.

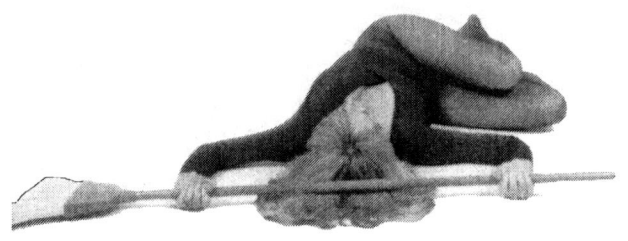

You are in competition with no one but your-self. The exercise is a tool to help smooth out those unwanted 'bumps.'

Always remember to:
♦ Press your upper spine and arms against the floor.
♦ Keep the arms at a 90 degree angle.
♦ Keep the knees pressed together.
♦ Inhale deeply, and twist as you <u>slowly</u> exhale.
♦ The slower the movements, the more isometric the exercise.
♦ Feel every muscle as you slowly 'twist' from side to side as far as YOU can.
♦ Visualize the side-to-side movements emanating from a central axis point in your lower back.
♦ As a finale:
stretch out, relax and visualize the results you will be reaping when you continue to do the
"5-way-twist".

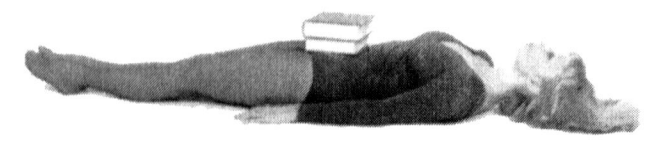

Here is another excellent exercise which helps make you more agile.

Follow my positions, alternating the legs into a stretch ... always **concentrate on pointing** the toes ... not only for good form, but to give your leg muscles an extra stretch.

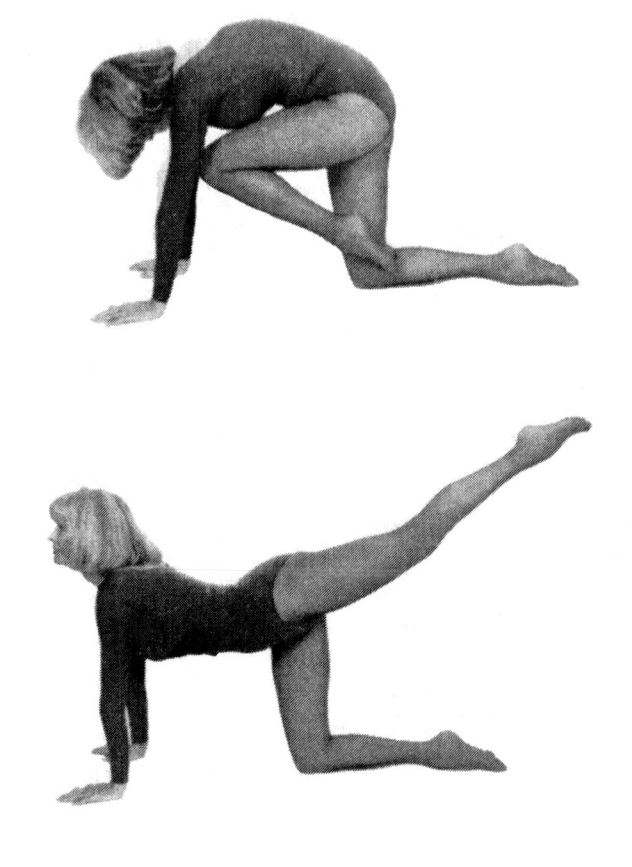

After stretching ... twisting ... and relaxing, follow my positions below... according to your agility. Remember, you will become more agile as you practice. So, don't give up if you feel stiff ... Rome was not built in one day!

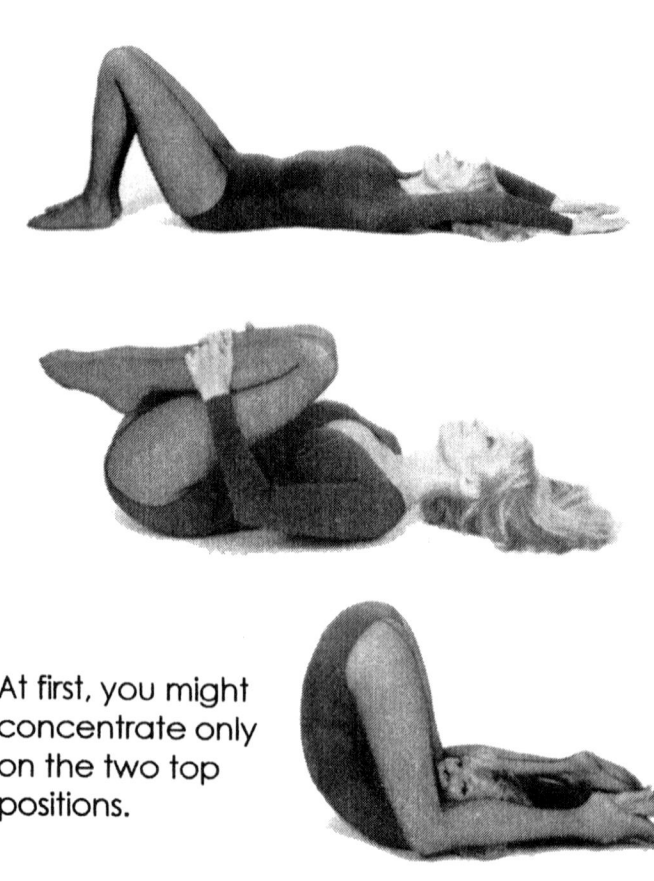

At first, you might concentrate only on the two top positions.

For beginners, all movements in this section should be repeated 5 to 10 times each ... add more at your own discretion.

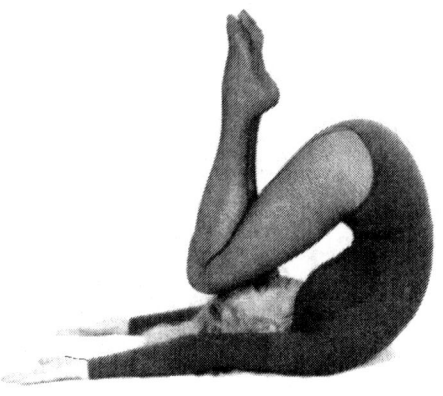

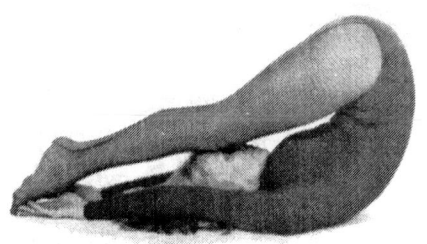

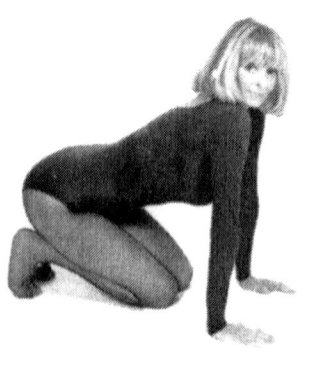

...and if you want to test your balance

try the **head stand**

remember ...
to clear the area!

Concentrate
on every move
and move slowly
to keep
your balance!

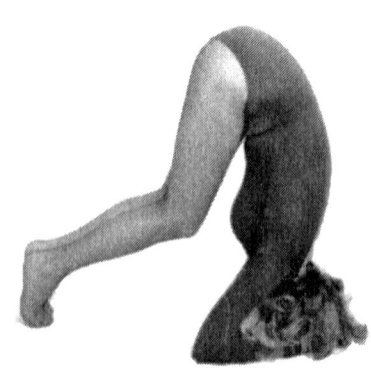

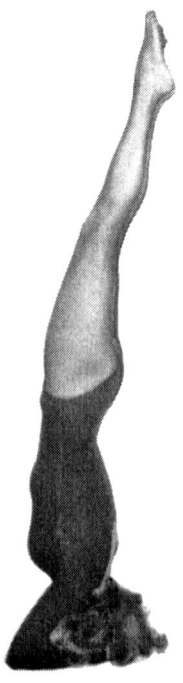

138

CHAPTER EIGHT

ANIMALS
HAVE RIGHTS TOO!

ANIMALS HAVE RIGHTS TOO!

It is always a pleasure to come home to my haven and be greeted by my roommate, a little fur person, who is most happy to see me. "Koschka" (cat in Russian), is a 14-year old ex-male cat, who was badly abused in his earlier years. When I rescued him, he was full of aggression and was ready to fight me off with every move I made. But after a few weeks he started to trust me, and became my shadow as he grew older. He let me employ him as a live heating pad – his loud purrs, which also act as a vibrator, indicate that he too enjoys his important position.

His soft, black and white fur often made me reflect on an area in Prague, which I passed while being taken for walks when I was a child. It was a building with large windows displaying, among other items ... pieces of black and white fur. At that time I could not understand what their use was, and was left with an uncomfortable feeling ... wondering what happened to the original owner of the fur.

Years later I found out that the fur was sold for the treatment of aches, general pains, and arthritis. Sadly, the originators of this 'treatment' were not aware that it is not the fur alone which helps in soothing ... it is a live, healthy, and trusting cat that will be only too happy to cooperate. The warmth and weight of the body, with the addition of vibrating purrs is the best heating/healing pad, I've ever found.

When cats feel secure and not threatened, they will take their 'heating pad' position very seriously.

I feel I have to add this sad and negative information ... which is a constant practice in research laboratories.

The unbelievable horrors of animal experimentation were visually impressed in my mind after visiting a large hospital in Washington D.C. where I observed the grotesque machinery and barbaric practices of medical doctors and their technicians. I shall never forget the sounds and sights of creatures whose stomachs were slit open and their intestines RIPPED OUT --- WHILE THEY WERE ALIVE AND CONSCIOUS! The tortured bodies were discarded in large garbage drums where the half dead creatures were trying desperately to claw their way out in a frenzy in their last fight from a painful and unnecessary death.

Large animals were strapped to walls and tables ... their eyes were filled with terror as they watched me ... in my own state of frozen horror when I realized what I was observing.

I truly can't understand how one still, in this age of advanced technology, can be programmed to believe that animals can be compared to our constitution and are still used in attempts to create cure-alls for many diseases, which are mostly created by mankind due to poor eating and drinking habits and inferior lifestyles.

If animal research is so successful, then why are all the diseases that afflict mankind still here ... even the simplest cold?! Instead, all these barbaric and costly energies could be directed to teaching children from the start how to live a healthy life based on good nutritional habits, good thoughts, sensitivity and productive habits.

I believe that junk food and sodas of all kind are the main cause of health problems ... they should be eliminated from the diet entirely ... **they are the beginning of the end.**

The self-indulgent need for instant gratification creates a culture of individuals who do not respect nature and its inhabitants, including themselves.

I think empathy, sensitivity and respect should be part of everyone's foundation and that starts with the creatures we are given charge of.

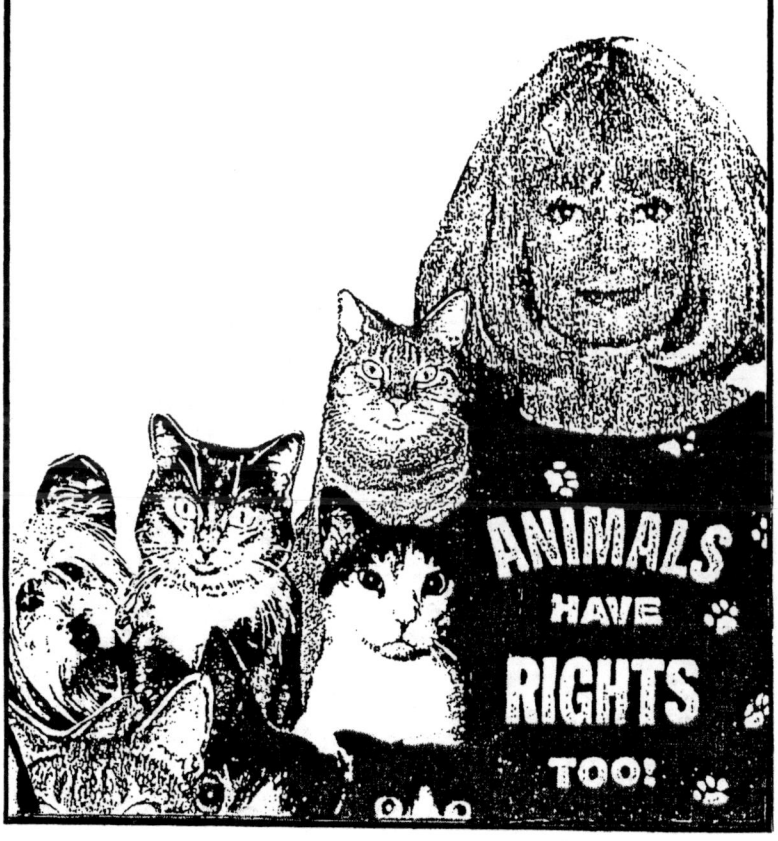

NOTES ...

IN CONCLUSION

<u>We are self-repairing ... all it takes:</u>

♥BELIEVE IN WHAT YOU DO♥

♥EAT THE RIGHT FOODS♥
and give your body a chance to change

♥EXERCISE ... OR TAKE A WALK♥
get stronger, more graceful and more agile

♥TRY TO THINK KIND THOUGHTS♥
and see the changes in your life

I hope this book
will be of help to you
and that you will
enjoy it ...
just as I have enjoyed
preparing it.

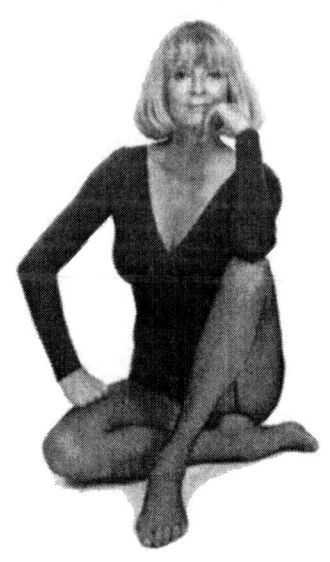

NOTES ...

OTHER BOOKS by Benita von Klingspor

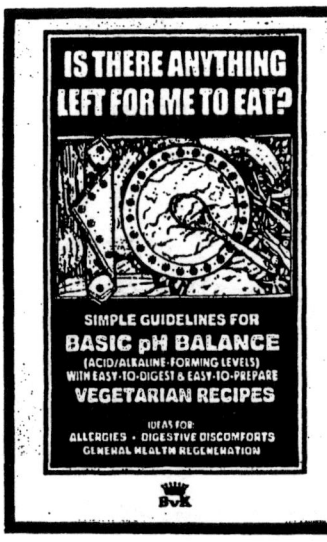

IS THERE ANYTHING
LEFT FOR ME TO EAT?

$14.95

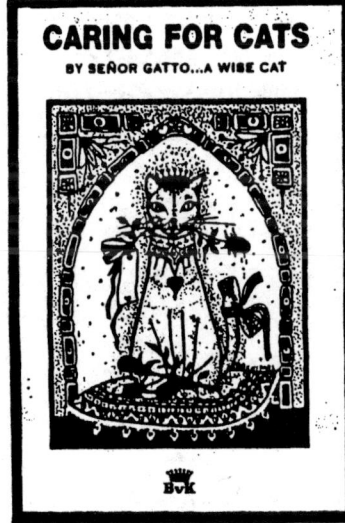

CARING FOR CATS

$12.95

◆ORDER FORM◆

TELEPHONE ORDERS:	(310) 578-5852		
POSTAL ORDERS:	BVK	P.O. BOX 9086	
	Marine del Rey, CA 90292		
E-MAIL:	benitaBVK@worldnet.att.net		

Please send me the following item(s):

TITLE	@ $	QU.	TOTAL
REJUVENATE!	16.95		
IS THERE ANYTHING LEFT FOR ME TO EAT?	14.95		
CARING FOR CATS	12.95		

SUB-TOTAL _____

TAX _____

S&H _____

TOTAL $ _____

SALES TAX: please add 8.25% for items shipped in California

SHIPPING: USA ... EACH BOOK $3.50 ... EACH ADDITIONAL $2.50

PAYMENT: MAIL CHECK TO: **BVK, P.O.BOX 9086**
MARINA DEL REY, CA-90292

YOUR NAME _____

ADDRESS _____

_____

_____

TELEPHONE_____

E-MAIL_____